Multiple Sclerosis

Multiple Sclerosis

UNDERSTANDING THE COGNITIVE CHALLENGES

. . . .

Nicholas LaRocca, PhD
Rosalind Kalb, PhD

WITH

John DeLuca, PhD
Lauren Caruso, PhD

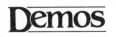

Demos Medical Publishing LLC
386 Park Avenue South, Suite 301
New York, NY 10016

Visit our website at www.demosmedpub.com

Library of Congress Cataloging-in-Publication Data
LaRocca, Nicholas.
  Multiple sclerosis : understanding the cognitive challenges / Nicholas LaRocca, Rosalind Kalb ; with John Deluca, Lauren Caruso.
    p. cm.
  Includes bibliographical references and index.
  ISBN-13: 978-1-932603-31-6 (alk. paper)
  ISBN-10: 1-932603-31-X (alk. paper)
  1. Multiple sclerosis—Complications—Popular works. 2. Cognition disorders—Popular works. I. Kalb, Rosalind. II. Title.
  RC377.L34 2006
  616.8'34—dc22

                                                          2006006253

Manufactured in the United States of America.

06 07 08 09 10   5 4 3 2 1

For everyone who has been affected by MS cognitive changes—with a special thank-you to those of you who have shared your struggles with us.

A Personal Note to the Reader

I n case you are wondering whether this book is for you, I'd like to give you a little encouragement to take the plunge. When I was diagnosed with MS in March of 1997, I cried because I immediately imagined myself unable to walk or do the things I love to do. When I began to have cognitive issues, I found myself wishing for those physical symptoms that had once seemed so frightening. If you have cognitive challenges, you know exactly what I mean. I wanted a disability that people could see, empathize with, and understand. I wanted them to know why I was having such a difficult time.

In the pages of this unique book, you will find that you are not alone. Although each person's experience with MS is different, you are likely to recognize yourself—your fears or challenges or solutions—in one or more of the chapters. You may even find yourself saying, "Wow—that sounds a lot like me."

I plan to share portions of this book with my family, friends, and colleagues. A lot of information is included here (that I have wanted to convey to them but haven't been able to put into my own words), which will help them better understand my daily challenges. I know that sharing this information with others will help me feel better about myself and reduce what I have come to call my "cognitive stress"—the reluctance I feel about entering into conversations for fear of losing my train of thought or making mistakes.

The book is well-written and easy to read. It makes the technical information more understandable and the personal issues less threatening. I encourage you to start by reading the authors' Preface. Their message is very comforting—like sitting in your favorite chair on a cold winter's night with a hot cup of cocoa. Then, I would suggest that you read the book in its entirety, share it with important people in your life when you are ready, and keep it close by as a reference guide.

Wishing you well,

Ann Borsellino

Contents

Foreword

As a neurologist specializing in the care of people with MS, I am well aware of the impact cognitive change can have on individuals and families and how frightening the possibility of cognitive dysfunction can be. This welcome addition to the MS literature invites those with concerns about MS-related cognitive change to exchange uncertainty and confusion for the information and strategies they need to get on with their lives. Multiple Sclerosis: Understanding the Cognitive Challenges lets people know that they are not alone—that other individuals and families are facing similar challenges and have found ways to manage and cope. With caring, warmth, and even subtle humor, the authors have made a difficult subject approachable and understandable.

Although relatively few of the 50% to 66% percent or so of people with MS who experience cognitive change will have to deal with major deficits, even mild changes can challenge one's self-confidence and impact daily life. For this reason, comprehensive yet understandable information about cognitive change is essential for individuals with MS, their family members, friends, and colleagues, and the health professionals involved in their care. This book provides useful definitions and a framework for thinking about the cognitive changes of MS, including an overview of the research findings gleaned since the mid 1990s, when this important topic emerged as a priority issue for those living with MS. The authors quickly dispel the long-held myth that there is nothing to be done about the cognitive symptoms of MS, providing information about ways to measure, treat, and compensate for changes that occur. In doing so, the authors—with extensive experience in MS clinical care and research—share with the reader their comforting optimism about the future of research and treatment in the area of cognition.

This unique book is thorough, current, and practical—offering a novel, hands-on approach to a difficult subject. It should be read not only by people with MS and their families, but also by general neurologists, primary care providers, and even MS specialists—neurologists and nurses. In fact, it should be read by any clinician providing care to individuals with multiple sclerosis.

The core messages contained in this book are important for all of us to remember. Like other possible symptoms of MS:

- Cognitive changes vary tremendously from one person to another—one size doesn't fit all.
- With proper diagnosis and assessment, cognitive changes can be managed.
- Changes in cognitive functioning must be understood and addressed within the total life framework of the person who is experiencing them. Simply understanding their relationship to MS and the damage it can cause to the brain is not enough; the emotional and social impact these changes can have needs to be understood by people with MS, their families and friends, and the health professionals who care for them.

The goal for everyone with MS is to function optimally and in the best of health. We have disease-modifying agents that deter progression. We have grappled with the physical symptoms of MS with a multitude of symptomatic treatments and a new generation of rehabilitation strategies.

We must now put a greater emphasis on tackling the cognitive issues. With this book—the very first of its kind—the authors point the way. The changes must be appreciated, recognized, and confronted by persons with MS and their health care professionals. As the authors point out, much progress has been made in identifying the changes that occur, educating people with MS and their families, building awareness among the medical community, and identifying treatment options. We must become better at putting this information to good use.

Linda Buchwald, MD

Preface

We have been asked many times over the years to write a book about cognition. The project seemed daunting for a variety of reasons, but primarily because we wanted to create a useful resource for people with MS and their family members—a resource that did justice to the complexity of the topic, yet was comprehensible and practical. Most of all, we wanted to help people feel more prepared to deal with the challenges that cognitive symptoms can cause in their work and personal lives. Feeling prepared generally starts with feeling informed, and it has been our mission in writing this book to provide information about many aspects of cognition in MS—when and how cognitive changes may occur; the ways in which these changes can impact a person emotionally, socially, and economically; the assessment tools that are used to diagnose and measure these changes; the treatment options to date; and some management strategies that can be used in everyday life.

Although it may feel easier and less frightening to put off thinking about MS-related cognitive changes, there are several important benefits to becoming informed about them as early as possible:

- Being knowledgeable about the ways in which MS can affect cognitive abilities will help you to recognize any problems you may be experiencing.
- Recognizing smaller problems before they become larger makes it easier to identify and implement treatments and management strategies.
- Having a better understanding of your cognitive challenges will enable you to explain them more clearly to important people in your life.

Chapter 1 describes what is meant by the term "cognition," and explains the four major functions that underlie our cognitive processes.

The second chapter is all about what it feels like to have one's ability to think, reason, and remember begin to change. We talk about the impact that cognitive changes can have on self-confidence and self-esteem, and on a person's relationships with family members, friends, and colleagues. Recognizing the stresses and strains that these symptoms can cause in different areas of one's life is the first step toward learning how to manage any changes that occur. The chapter lists important strategies for minimizing the impact of cognitive change on one's personal and professional life—all of which are explained in greater detail in the remainder of the book.

Chapter 3 offers a comprehensive overview of what we know— and don't know—about cognition and MS. For some, this will be exactly the kind of in-depth review of the relevant research that you have been waiting for, complete with a list of references to provide you with even more information. For others, this chapter may be the one you choose to read last—after you have read all about the ways in which your own cognitive symptoms might be identified, measured, treated, and managed. In other words, you may be more interested in how all this applies to you and your family than to the MS world at large.

The fourth chapter of the book discusses how cognitive changes might look and feel to those who are living with them, and describes the types of formal assessments that can be done to identify those areas of cognition that have been affected by MS and those that remain unchanged. This is particularly important because the areas of cognitive function that remain strong become valuable tools to help compensate for areas that have been compromised in some way.

Chapter 5 is all about treatment options—what the research suggests may be useful and what not—while Chapter 6 offers some ideas for managing any cognitive changes that you might be experiencing. The goal is to provide you with instructions and easy-to-follow examples that will enable you to develop personalized strategies to fit your style, abilities, and situation.

The last chapter presents a series of vignettes. The goal of these vignettes is to provide snapshots of individual lives that have been impacted by cognitive changes, along with examples of the kinds of compensatory strategies that can make these changes more manageable. While you are unlikely to find anyone in this book—or in a support group or chat room—whose situation is exactly like yours, it is our hope that *Multiple Sclerosis: Understanding the Cognitive*

Challenges will at least help you feel less alone in your efforts to manage the cognitive symptoms of MS.

The book ends with a glossary of terms, including all those words in the text that appear in bold italics.

A central message of this book is that cognitive symptoms—like all the possible symptoms of MS—vary tremendously from one person to another. If you are among the 50% to 66% or so of people with MS who experience cognitive changes, there is no detailed roadmap to follow. The key to managing the changes that occur will lie in tapping the appropriate resources—to get the problem accurately identified and adequately measured, to utilize whichever treatment interventions you and your physician agree would be best for you, to develop the management strategies that work most effectively for your particular symptoms and lifestyle, and to keep tweaking them if and when your needs change.

We hope that this book will help guide you along the way.

CHAPTER **I**

WHAT IS COGNITION?

John DeLuca, PhD

●●

It is fairly common to hear people with multiple sclerosis (MS) complain of problems remembering things, finding the right words, concentrating on a task or something they are reading, or following a conversation. Often, a person with MS will joke with family and friends about such "MS moments," although deep inside, he or she is not really laughing. "Am I going crazy?" or "Am I losing my mind?" are not uncommon questions, especially in one's private thoughts.[1]

The dictionary broadly defines *cognition* as "the act or process of knowing." More specifically, cognitive functions can be compared to the computer's operations of input, storage, processing, and output. Thus, cognition can be divided into four general areas:

- Receptive functions, including (a) integrating input from the five senses, (b) paying attention, (c) rapidly processing incoming information from the environment, and (d) selecting and classifying that incoming information
- Learning and memory, including (a) acquiring new information, (b) storing the information, and (c) retrieving it when needed
- Thinking, which is the mental organization and manipulation of information
- Execution and expressive functions, which include acting upon and communicating information to others[2]

Cognition should be distinguished from emotions (one's feelings and motivations) and from personality (one's distinctive or personal

2

characteristics). In reality, however, such divisions are artificial—we have created them for our own convenience. In other words, just as we divide a functioning body into seemingly separate systems (immune, skeletal, nervous, etc.), in reality, the systems all work together to form the human self.

For example, if one has difficulty following conversations in public because of slowed information-processing speed, or has difficulty finding the right word while speaking to others, this "cognitive" dysfunction can cause the person to feel "stupid" and "out of place," which in turn can lead to feelings of embarrassment and concerns about looking inadequate in the eyes of others. Such thoughts and feelings can lead to social withdrawal, feelings of depression, and "personality change," as we will talk about later in this book. Thus, understanding the "division" between cognition, emotions, and personality—and the interplay among these factors—is an important part of understanding the influence that MS can have on behavior and one's sense of self.

References

1. Hall K. About...um...I forgot!! *InsideMS* 1999;17:52–53.
2. Lezak MD. *Neuropsychological Assessment*, 3rd ed. New York: Oxford University Press, 1995.

CHAPTER **2**

THE EMOTIONAL AND SOCIAL IMPACT OF COGNITIVE CHANGES

Rosalind Kalb, PhD

• •

Problems with thinking and memory can have a profound impact on a person's self-image and self-esteem, as well as on his or her relationships with others. Adapting to changes in oneself and finding ways to communicate about them to others can be a significant challenge. Recognizing the stresses and strains these symptoms can cause is the first step in learning how to cope with and manage any changes that occur. This chapter describes the emotional and social challenges that can result from multiple sclerosis (MS)-related cognitive changes, and provides some strategies for meeting these challenges.

THE POTENTIAL IMPACT OF COGNITIVE SYMPTOMS ON PERSONAL IDENTITY AND SELF-ESTEEM

The ability to think, remember, and reason is central to who we are. Even more than our physical abilities, these cognitive processes define us as individuals, unique from everyone else. When our cognition is threatened or changed in any way, we tend to feel somewhat lost and confused—as though we had misplaced the person we relied on and now have to get reacquainted with someone slightly different.

Changes in cognitive abilities can cause people to lose their self-confidence, feel "stupid," or become chronically anxious about "messing up" or "looking foolish." Particularly for someone whose sense of identity and self-worth is highly dependent on intellectual rather than physical functioning, even the slightest changes in cognitive abilities can be very frightening.

A person who is experiencing significant physical changes as a result of MS may also see cognitive changes as "adding insult to injury." Having already begun to deal with the fact that his or her body is no longer functioning the way it used to, the person may resist or deny the possibility that MS can also affect the mind. Reluctance to accept the possibility of MS-related cognitive changes is one of the factors that cause many people to delay discussing the problems with their doctor or seeking out an evaluation.

WAYS IN WHICH COGNITIVE CHANGES CAN IMPACT A PERSON'S SENSE OF SELF

A person's sense of self is made up of many parts. Among the most important are confidence in one's ability to perform adequately in chosen roles (self-confidence) and a positive feeling about one's value as a person (self-esteem). The following are examples of ways in which cognitive challenges can impact feelings of self-confidence and self-esteem:

- **Carrying out familiar routines:** Difficulty in remembering, organizing, or implementing familiar routines at home or at work can shake a person's confidence in his or her capabilities and interfere with the pleasurable rhythms of daily life. Without the comfort provided by familiar routines, a person begins to doubt his or her ability to manage activities and contribute meaningfully at work and at home.

- **Remembering recent conversations or activities:** The inability to remember the details of recent conversations or activities can leave a person feeling disoriented, disconnected, and empty—as though "holes" now exist in his or her life. Worry and embarrassment about this kind of memory problem can lead someone to avoid interactions and become increasingly isolated.

- **Thinking clearly and smoothly:** When thought processes feel slowed or stuck, the person may be left feeling immobilized—unable to hold on to incoming information, respond appropriately, or make effective decisions. When the ability to respond adequately to incoming information is altered, a person may begin to feel less in control and increasingly disconnected from a world that is moving much too fast.

- **Finding the right word:** People who have problems finding words (the tip-of-the tongue phenomenon) may feel embarrassed, misunderstood, anxious about talking to others, and afraid of misspeaking or saying something wrong. Concerns about one's ability to communicate effectively with others may cause a person to avoid social situations, leading to increasing isolation.

- **Maintaining focus and attention:** A person who has difficulty maintaining focus without getting distracted may experience disruptions in many of the pleasurable activities of daily life, including reading or watching TV, carrying on meaningful conversations with other people, and maintaining arousal during sexual activity. The same inability to maintain focus can interfere with tasks at home and reduce one's effectiveness at work, significantly impacting feelings of self-worth.

- **Maintaining a sense of visual-spatial orientation and spatial relationships:** Problems with spatial orientation can result in getting lost and feeling disoriented in any but the most familiar surroundings, leading a person to feel fearful about driving a car or venturing out of his neighborhood. This can result in a loss of social contacts if that person has no alternative means of transportation. People who experience difficulties in this area can also lose confidence in their ability to build or assemble objects or follow directions for doing this kind of assembly.

- **Planning and problem solving:** People who have difficulty organizing their thoughts, prioritizing and planning their activities, or identify the sequence of steps needed to solve a problem or complete an activity may become overwhelmed and surrounded by uncompleted tasks. A person with problems in this area—particularly someone who has always taken pride in his or her organizational skills and productivity—may begin to feel ineffective, immobilized, and out or control.

STRATEGIES FOR REBUILDING FEELINGS OF CONFIDENCE AND SELF-ESTEEM

Healthy Grieving

As with any other change or loss caused by MS, it is important to allow yourself to grieve over the cognitive changes that occur. Grief is a normal reaction to changes over which we have no control, and cognitive problems are no exception. Healthy grieving sets the stage for adaptive coping and problem-solving by allowing you to let go of "the way things used to be" and preparing you to think about ways to do things differently in the future. The self-confidence and self-esteem that have been threatened or lost because of the cognitive symptoms you are experiencing are regained as you put in place strategies to compensate for the changes and get on with your important life activities.

Education

Becoming educated about MS-related cognitive problems will enable you to understand what is happening and why. This type of understanding is important for three reasons: First, it makes the changes more comprehensible and less frightening; as with any other symptoms of MS, you will then feel more prepared to explore treatment options. Second, it can help reduce feelings of inadequacy, self-blame, and guilt. Last, it will help prepare you to explain the changes to others. Chapter 3 provides a detailed review of the research that has been done on cognition in MS. Additional information about MS-related cognitive dysfunction is available from a variety of sources, including books, journal articles, pamphlets from the National Multiple Sclerosis Society, and Web-based, learn-online programs sponsored by the Society.

Cognitive Assessment

When cognitive changes occur, people have a tendency to feel as if they are "losing it," "becoming stupid," or "getting senile." A cognitive evaluation by a trained professional (neuropsychologist, occupational therapist, or speech-language pathologist) will give you a more specific and accurate picture of what is going on. It will enable you to pinpoint the changes that have occurred and develop a clearer understanding of how these changes impact everyday activities. The assessment will also highlight your areas of strength and weakness—information that will be critical as you look for ways to manage your cognitive challenges. Your strengths will be the tools you use to compensate for any areas of weakness. Utilizing your strengths will not only enhance your functioning in everyday life, but will help you regain your confidence and self-esteem as well. Chapter 4 describes the assessment process in detail, whereas Chapter 6 provides examples of compensatory strategies that can be used to manage daily activities that have been disrupted by cognitive changes.

The brief vignettes in Chapter 7 demonstrate how some individuals have utilized the information from their cognitive assessments to develop effective compensatory strategies.

Cognitive Remediation

Working with a trained professional on a regular basis to identify tools and strategies to compensate for cognitive changes is a further step toward rebuilding your confidence. Chapter 5 provides a review of the research that has been done on various treatment options, and discusses the remediation process in detail. Your neurologist, MS center, or chapter of the National Multiple Sclerosis Society can refer you to qualified professionals in your area.

Emotional Support

As with any other aspects of living with MS, you may find that you need the support and encouragement of others—particularly people who are experiencing similar kinds of challenges. People with MS often say that it is important to be able to talk with others who "get it"—who know what the various symptoms of MS can feel like, and who have identified strategies to deal with them. If you are not comfortable in a support group setting, you can also find support with an individual counselor or in chat rooms and bulletin boards on the Internet (although care must be taken to choose websites carefully and verify information with an MS professional).

Educate Others

With or without the help of a professional counselor, it will be important to share information about your cognitive challenges—and the strategies you are using to manage them—with those closest to you. This will help dispel any misunderstandings that have developed around your symptoms and ensure that the lines of communication are open. You might, for example, explain your difficulties by giving specific examples of cognitive tasks that have begun to give you difficulty in daily life. Or, you might invite your spouse/partner or close friend to come with you to the feedback session following your cognitive evaluation, or share the report that you receive. Like any "invisible" symptom of MS (fatigue or pain, for example), cognitive changes can be very difficult for others to understand—and you need to be prepared to explain and explain and explain again.

Once family members and friends have an understanding of what is occurring and why, they can be invaluable allies in your efforts to deal with cognitive symptoms. As their understanding of the changes grows, they will be in an ideal position to provide emotional and practical support for the compensatory strategies you are using. Being able to fulfill your responsibilities and maintain your role within the household is a major step toward regaining your confidence and self-esteem.

If you find that others tend to dismiss what you are telling them (e.g., "Oh, that happens to me all the time..." "We're all getting older you know..." "We all know what that's like..."), you may find it useful to share with them some written information about MS-related cognitive dysfunction. The National Multiple Sclerosis Society has brochures and Web-based materials on cognition that will help others understand what you are talking about. The important thing is to recognize that most of these people are trying to be reassuring and supportive; with the appropriate information and education from you, they will soon catch on to what you are telling them.

THE POTENTIAL IMPACT OF COGNITIVE CHANGES ON FAMILY RELATIONSHIPS

Changes in cognitive abilities can impact long-standing relationships and disrupt family life. Because the changes tend to develop slowly and insidiously, they are often poorly understood—both by the person who is experiencing them and by family members and friends. It is easy for a spouse, partner, or child to misinterpret problems with attention or memory, for example as "You're not listening...." "You don't care enough to pay attention or remember...." "You're getting stupid...."—or problems with organization as "You have gotten so sloppy...." or "You can't seem to keep track of anything...!"

Here are some examples of ways in which cognitive changes can impact family relationships:

- Feelings of resentment can arise when the person with MS feels that he or she has a cognitive challenge that family members deny or dismiss, or when the person with MS denies having a problem that family members recognize and try to talk about.
- Cognitive changes can alter the balance in relationships. Spouses or partners may feel that their "equal" partnership is becoming less equal, as the well partner has to take on more of the family and household responsibilities. Children, particularly teenagers,

may try to take advantage of a parent's memory problems to get their own way. Children of all ages may feel pressure to take on a more protective role.

- A spouse, partner, or child may begin to doubt the abilities, competence, or judgment of the person with MS ("I can't count on this person any more"), thus affecting his or her confidence in, or respect for, that person.

- Memory and attention problems can affect interpersonal communication in ways that make conversations slower, more repetitive, less interesting, and less productive. Family members become frustrated at being asked the same questions repeatedly and having to repeat the same answers over and over again. The person with MS who has difficulty remembering conversations may begin to feel "out of the loop" and disconnected from family communications.

- Cognitive problems (e.g., impaired memory, organizational skills, and information processing) can disrupt daily activities and routines in ways that alter the long-standing rhythms of the household, making daily life feel less predictable and more chaotic.

- Family members who become anxious about the welfare of the person who gets lost easily, doesn't remember to do things like turn off the stove or lock the door, goes through red lights or misses other cues while driving, or demonstrates impulsivity or impaired judgment, often feel the need to monitor or supervise their loved one. This alteration in roles tends to shift the balance of family relationships, thereby impacting virtually every aspect of family life.

STRATEGIES FOR MANAGING COGNITIVE CHANGES WITH FAMILY MEMBERS

Education

Keep in mind that less visible symptoms are much harder for family members to see and understand. Both spouses/partners and children have reported that the cognitive changes caused by MS are among the most difficult symptoms to understand and accept. "This isn't the same person" is a fairly common refrain. By explaining to family members (including your children) what you are experiencing and how they can be of help, you are taking a major step toward managing your symptoms, relieving everyone's anxiety, and getting the family system back on track. You may find it useful to share with family members the results of your cognitive evaluation, and/or invite them to a joint meeting with the professional who has done the evaluation. This will give them an ideal opportunity to ask questions, increase their understanding of your cognitive symptoms, and share any concerns they may have.

Family Problem-Solving

Your family members can help you (and the cognitive remediation specialist, if you are working with one) identify strategies to manage cognitive challenges around the house. They may, for example, be able to suggest ways for everyone in the household to help with organization, with tracking everyone's busy schedules on a family calendar, or with strategies for recording phone messages in a consistent place. When you engage family members in brainstorming about problem-solving strategies, you enhance their understanding of the challenges you face and go a long way toward helping them help you.

Family Involvement in Compensatory Strategies

Be sure to involve family members in any compensatory strategies that your cognitive rehabilitation specialist has recommended for you. For these strategies to work effectively, you need buy-in from those around you. For example, developing organizational strategies to help you remember where things are kept in the house won't work unless others in the house cooperate by putting any items they use back where they belong. Working to minimize environmental distractions during conversations, so that you can process and remember what people are saying, won't be effective if others don't do their part—for example, by turning off the TV or radio.

Maintaining Family Patterns

All families develop a rhythm and structure of their own. When the familiar patterns of daily life give way to chaos, no one is comfortable. To the extent that you can maintain these patterns in spite of MS-related changes, you will help to reduce uncertainty and relieve anxiety. Even though you may need the help and support of your children, for example, it is important for you—and them—to remember who is in charge. Even if it takes you longer to do some of the things you have to do, or you need to trade chores and responsibilities with other family members, you can maintain your position in the family by managing and coordinating these changes.

Professional Counseling

If communicating with family members about any of these changes becomes too difficult, or you encounter more resistance than feels manageable, you may want to seek help from a family counselor. Sometimes it takes professional assistance to jump-start the communication process.

Reacting to Family Members' Concerns

It happens occasionally that family members become aware of MS-related cognitive changes before the person with MS is able to recognize or acknowledge them. If your family members begin to express concerns about your memory, or your organizational or driving abilities, for example, your first reaction may be to deny, argue, or simply get angry. It is never easy to be confronted with this kind of information, even by the people you love most. Try to keep in mind, however, that those closest to you are also the people who are most concerned about your well-being. If you don't feel ready to hear or discuss what they have to say, try telling them that you appreciate their concern and will give it some thought. Simply brushing them off is only likely to make them push harder.

Take some time to read about MS-related cognitive changes, discuss them with your doctor, and consider honestly whether you might be experiencing any problems. When you feel prepared to handle the conversation, begin by asking your family members what they have noticed and what their concerns are. Your willingness to engage in this kind of conversation will reassure them while also giving a clear message that you are taking steps to manage your MS symptoms. This is the beginning of effective problem-solving.

HOW COGNITIVE CHANGES CAN IMPACT RELATIONSHIPS AT WORK AND SCHOOL

Our roles at work or school help to define who we are. Because they involve a significant amount of time, effort, and energy, these roles contribute to our feelings of accomplishment, satisfaction, and pride. In other words, activities at work or school are central to a person's self-image and self-esteem. Cognitive symptoms can interfere with work-related activities just as physical impairments can—only the changes can be more difficult to pinpoint and manage. Less visible changes may also be more difficult for employers, colleagues, teachers, and fellow students to understand and accept. Quite understandably, people with MS are often more reluctant to talk about cognitive difficulties with non-family members—particularly since the ability to succeed in educational and vocational arenas has major long-term implications—emotionally, financially, and socially.

Cognitive changes can interfere with activities and relationships at work or school in a variety of ways:

- Problems with memory, information processing, and attention can interfere with a person's ability to acquire and retain new information and skills—both of which are essential to growth and success.
- Attentional problems can lead to errors, which are easily misunderstood by others as carelessness, disinterest, or lack of requisite skills.
- Changes in executive functions, including organization, prioritizing, and planning and problem-solving, can interfere with the timely initiation and completion of tasks—which can diminish the confidence and respect of others.
- Word-finding problems and slowed processing speed can impact interpersonal communication and be misinterpreted as lack of ability or understanding.
- Cognitive changes that reduce performance can easily be misunderstood by employers and colleagues as incompetence, lack of interest, inattention, emotional problems, or drug or alcohol abuse.

In addition, cognitive changes that interfere with job performance can affect a person's sense of self-worth and confidence in his or her abilities. Someone who is used to having a significant impact in the workplace can begin to feel worthless and unnecessary, which in turn will make it more difficult to perform and interact comfortably with others.

Strategies for Managing Cognitive Changes at Work or School

Cognitive changes and fatigue are the most common reasons why people with MS leave the workforce. Sometimes this early retirement is by choice; other times it is not. Your primary goal should be to remain employed as long as you are interested and able to do so. A complete discussion of strategies to maintain employment would go far beyond the scope of this book. In relation to cognitive changes, however, your primary goal should be to recognize the challenges you are having before your employer or colleagues do. (See Chapter 4 for a discussion of ways to recognize cognitive changes.)

Sharing information about cognitive problems in the workplace is very different from sharing it with family members or close friends because disclosure to one's manager has potentially major implications for your professional future and financial well-being. It will be well worth your while to think carefully about how much to tell your employer and colleagues about any cognitive difficulties you are having; once this information has been given, there is no way to take it back. Because this is such an important decision, we urge you to consult with your National Multiple Sclerosis Society chapter and/or vocational counselor or disability attorney to ensure that you are aware of your options and their potential implications. Your decision will depend on the types of problems you are experiencing, the kind of setting in which you work, your relationships with your manager and co-workers, and your own needs for privacy or openness.

If you determine that certain types of accommodations within the workplace—such as flex-time, a brief rest period in the afternoon, or a particular type of computer software, for example—would help you be more effective in your job, you can explain that you have a disability for which these types of accommodations would be helpful. Although you may be reluctant to disclose that you have a disability, keep in mind that an employer is far more likely to retain confidence in an employee who recognizes and addresses a challenge before it becomes a problem than one who waits until the problems have already had a negative impact on the office or company.

Resources are listed at the end of this chapter to help you understand and implement the job-accommodation process. In the meantime, it probably doesn't do you or your co-workers any good to talk at length about memory or organizational problems you are having.

If, after careful consideration, you decide that it would be more comfortable to have an in-depth conversation with your employer about your cognitive symptoms, your best strategy is to begin by educating him or her about MS-related cognitive dysfunction. The next step is to explain how your particular symptoms affect your job, and what strategies you have already identified to deal with them. Again, you are taking a proactive role in addressing the problems so that your employer doesn't have to.

The same kinds of cognitive symptoms that can affect one's performance at work can also have an impact on academic performance. Although one doesn't run the risk of being "fired" from school, there is the obvious risk of doing poorly or not graduating. Fortunately, most colleges and universities now offer accommodations for students with special needs. Equipped with a note from your physician explaining that you have a disability, and a list of the accommodations you need (preferably provided by a cognitive remediation specialist) to succeed in the school environment, you will usually be able to get the necessary accommodations (e.g., permission to bring a tape recorder into class, untimed testing, a quiet room in which to take a test, open-book testing).

Cognitive remediation specialists can work with you to identify on-the-job or school-related compensatory techniques. Enhancing your organizational strategies, for example, can help compensate for memory impairments. The more organized you are, the less you need to rely on your memory to tell you when to do things, where to put important papers, what's next on your schedule.

As with every other aspect of MS, no two people will experience cognitive changes in exactly the same way, and many people won't experience them at all. Therefore, no chapter in a book can capture every person's challenges or describe all the various ways in which a person's symptoms might affect life at home or out in the world. In this chapter, we have provided examples to help you identify the ways in which cognitive changes might be affecting you and your relationships with important people in your life, and we have suggested strategies to help you navigate these changes as effectively and comfortably as possible. Your individual issues may be best explored and addressed by working with a cognitive specialist who can provide a comprehensive assessment and make appropriate treatment recommendations.

The next chapter provides an overview of what research on cognition has been able to teach us about the changes that people with MS—as a group—may experience. It defines the many functions that make the human mind so complex, and identifies those functions that are most likely to be affected by MS and those that tend to remain unchanged. The chapter also explains what we know about the relationship between cognitive changes and other aspects of the disease. Like any other overview of research findings, it provides a snapshot of available knowledge. Because every person with MS is unique, and each person's disease course is unpredictable, you may find yourself in that snapshot or you may not. The goal is to provide you with an overview of the current knowledge in the field and the opportunity to read further in the research literature if you choose to do so.

Additional Resources

RECOMMENDED READING FROM DEMOS MEDICAL PUBLISHING

Kalb R (ed.). *Multiple Sclerosis: The Questions You Have; The Answers You Need*, 3rd ed., 2004.
   Ch. 9 Cognition—LaRocca N, Sorensen, P
   Ch. 10 Psychosocial Issues—Kalb R, Miller D
   Ch. 14 Employment—Rumrill P, Hennessey M
Kalb R (ed.). *Multiple Sclerosis: A Guide for Families*, 3rd ed., 2005.
   Ch. 2 Emotional and Cognitive Issues—LaRocca N

INFORMATION FROM THE NATIONAL MULTIPLE SCLEROSIS SOCIETY

For answers to questions about MS and its management, contact the National Multiple Sclerosis Society at 1-800-FIGHT-MS (1-800-344-4867), or visit the Society's website at www.nationalmssociety.org.
Publications also are available by calling 1-800-FIGHT-MS or online in the:
   Library section of the website (www.nationalmssociety.org/Brochures)
   Web Spotlight on Cognition (www.nationalmssociety.org/Cognition)
   Web Spotlight on Employment (www.nationalmssociety.org/Employment)

CHAPTER 3

WHAT WE KNOW ABOUT COGNITIVE CHANGES IN MULTIPLE SCLEROSIS

John DeLuca, PhD

• •

In this chapter, we review what the research studies over the past several years have been able to tell us about multiple sclerosis (MS)-related cognitive changes. References have been included for those who are interested in reading the original studies in greater detail.

HOW COMMON IS COGNITIVE DYSFUNCTION IN MS?

Only a few decades ago *cognitive impairment* was considered rare among people with MS—present in perhaps only 3% of the MS population. However, with the use of more sophisticated neuropsychologic evaluations and techniques, it is now well known that 50%–66% of people with MS have some level of cognitive problems.[1] Consider that, for over 100 years, people with MS have suffered with the frustrations and distress of simply trying to describe their cognitive problems to their doctors, family members, and friends, only to hear that "You are just depressed," or "MS does not cause cognitive problems," or "We're all getting older."

Today, MS specialists are fully aware that MS can result in significant cognitive impairment. These cognitive difficulties can range from mild to moderate to severe in degree, with the highest prevalence in the mild-moderate range. Nonetheless, it is also now clear that the presence of such cognitive impairments can have significant consequences on a person's ability to function comfortably. It also should be recognized that, with proper understanding and professional attention, cognitive problems can be managed in ways that minimize their interference in everyday life. Because cognitive impairments can be frightening and disruptive for oneself, one's family, and others, it is important to discuss concerns about cognition with your physician and seek the proper professional (usually a neuropsychologist, occupational therapist, or speech-language pathologist) to help deal with the challenges that these impairments bring to everyday life.

WHAT ARE THE COGNITIVE PROBLEMS ASSOCIATED WITH MS?

In a nutshell, the overall cognitive problem in MS could be described as a reduction in mental "sharpness." The major areas of cognition that can be impaired in MS are listed in Table 3.1.

More than 30 years of neuropsychologic research have been able to delineate specific impairments that can be associated with MS. It is important to note, however, that MS is a highly variable illness; not all people with MS will display all of these cognitive problems, and no two people will experience exactly the same types or severity of problems. Just as the nature, frequency, and severity of MS-related physical problems can vary across individuals, the same is

TABLE 3.1. Cognitive functioning in people with MS

Often impaired:
    Complex attention (e.g., multitasking)
    Information-processing speed
    Learning and memory
    Perceptual skills
    Executive functions (e.g., problem solving, initiation, organization, planning)
    Word finding
Usually intact:
    Basic attention
    Essential verbal skills (comprehension, expression, naming, repetition)
    Intelligence

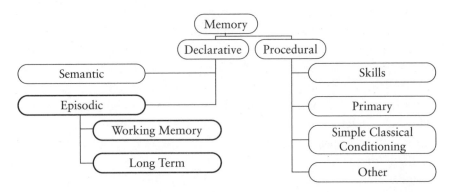

FIGURE 3.1. Structure of the memory system. Boxes with dark border indicate memory functions that may be affected in MS. Adapted with permission from Squire LR. *Memory and Brain.* New York: Oxford University Press, 1987.

true of a person's cognitive profile. This heterogeneity among people with MS must be kept in mind when reading the following overview.

Learning and Memory

Problems with memory are the most frequent complaint among people with MS and those that have received the greatest research attention. A review of memory studies shows that approximately 40% of people with MS have either no memory impairments or very mild ones; 30% show moderate impairment, and 30% have severe difficulty.[2]

Learning and memory interact in a very complex way. Although they are often discussed as a single entity, learning and memory consist of multiple levels and processes (Figure 3.1).[3] At its broadest level, memory can be divided into ***declarative memory*** (conscious recollection of facts, knowledge, experiences, and events) and ***procedural memory***, which refers to sensory-motor and skill-based learning (i.e., the knowledge of how to perform activities such as riding a bike or playing the piano). Procedural memory is not necessarily accessible to conscious experience or recollection. Procedural memory is generally intact in people with MS. Declarative memory can be further subdivided into ***episodic memory*** and ***semantic memory***. Episodic memory refers to memory for events, facts, and experiences that have occurred (e.g., recalling the name of your second-grade teacher). Semantic memory reflects general knowledge and the recognition and meaning of words, objects, actions, and facts that are not tied to a specific time and place of learning (such as the meaning of vocabulary words). Semantic memory is generally not affected in people with MS.

So, the learning and memory problem in those with MS lies primarily within episodic memory, which itself can be divided into *working memory* (which used to be called short-term memory) and *long-term memory*. Working memory (WM) refers to the short-term storage (up to 15 or 20 seconds) of information, as well as the mental manipulation of this stored information. It is the process that keeps information active or "in mind." For example, if one were to add the numbers 5 + 3, each number would need to be stored long enough to perform the mental manipulation of adding them together. Good research evidence suggests that people with MS have difficulty with WM, particularly during the mental manipulation portion.

Long-term memory (LTM) refers to information that has been considered sufficiently important to be stored in the brain "indefinitely," for later retrieval. If WM has to do with the short-term, temporary storage and manipulation of material, then all other episodic recall is part of LTM. As such, although it is common to consider the recall of recent information (e.g., what one had for breakfast) as part of short-term (or WM) memory, this is actually not the case. If considered "important," it will be entered into LTM for indefinite storage.

It is also possible to divide LTM into *retrograde memory*, which refers to recall of information stored before damage to the brain, and *anterograde memory*, which refers to the recall of newly learned information. In general, people with MS do not have a problem with retrograde memory (i.e., recalling the name of your second-grade teacher). Thus, the major impairment in people with MS is in acquiring and remembering new information.

As is evident here, one way to understand the complexity of human learning and memory is to become familiar with its various components. Another approach that helps in understanding memory dysfunction is to examine the "process" by which memory becomes impaired. This "information processing" approach looks to determine where in the process of memory formation the performance breaks down. In this model, memory formation can be divided into the *acquisition phase* and the *retrieval phase* (Figure 3.2). Acquisition refers to the gathering of information or "the sensory uptake of information, its initial encoding, and further consolidation (or storing information in the brain)."[4] Retrieval refers to the recall of that information, or "the process of recovering previously encoded (and stored) information."[5]

Dividing the memory process into acquisition versus retrieval mechanisms allows for the examination of where in the learning and

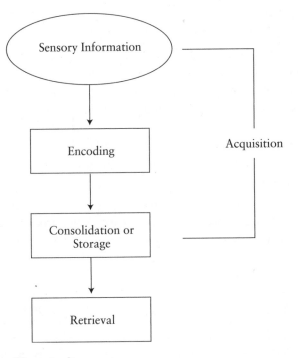

FIGURE 3.2. The episodic memory process.

memory process a person is experiencing difficulty. For example, is the person having difficulty in the initial learning of information or does the difficulty lie in the retrieval of information from long-term storage? This process approach has been particularly useful in studying the nature of learning and memory impairments in people with MS.

Until recently, it was generally thought that people with MS experienced impairments in the retrieval of information from long-term storage in the brain. This "retrieval hypothesis" suggested that people with MS had no trouble learning information and storing it appropriately in the brain. Rather, the core deficit involved problems retrieving that information from storage. However, more recent research suggests this is not the case. This newer research has shown that people with MS have difficulty primarily in the learning or acquisition of information rather than in retrieval.[6–9]

This recent finding is very important for people with MS. It suggests that factors that decrease one's ability to adequately learn new information may have a significant impact on one's ability to remember it later. These factors can be other cognitive functions (described below), such as difficulties in attention/concentration, working memory, perceptual skills, speed of information processing or executive functions, or other factors such as lack of sleep, MS-related fatigue, medication side effects, depression or anxiety, or just "having a bad day." Another important implication of this new research is that, once information has been adequately learned, people with MS will forget that information at the same rate as do individuals without MS. This, in itself, should be comforting news for anyone with MS.

One advantage of an information-processing approach to the study of impaired memory is that the findings have significant implications for rehabilitation and treatment. Treatment for problems with the acquisition of new information will focus on techniques to improve learning, although treatment for problems with retrieval of information would rely more on techniques to aid in the search for stored memories.

Information Processing

Like most cognitive skills, the ability to process information is very complex. It all starts with adequate sensory input—something that is not guaranteed in people with MS. For example, many people with MS experience visual impairments from optic neuritis, which may alter the processing of incoming visual information. The next step after sensory input is adequate attention. Whereas some studies clearly demonstrate problems with attention, people with MS generally have little difficulty focusing their attention on given tasks. They experience greater difficulty in sustaining that attention over time (which may result in cognitive fatigue[10] (see p. 32); or in dividing their attention among several tasks simultaneously (also referred to as "multitasking").

By far, the most significant information processing problem among people with MS is the speed with which cognitive information is processed. Several studies have clearly demonstrated slowed information-processing speed in people with MS.[11–15] For example, one study found that slowed processing speed is 10 times more likely to be observed among people with MS than in the general population, and this occurrence increases to 65 times more among people with secondary-progressive MS.[12] Another study showed that people with MS were 40% slower than healthy control subjects on tasks of processing speed.[16]

Recent research has been interested in answering the following question: Is impaired performance on tests of processing speed due to a reduced ability to process information, or is it a function of impaired accuracy? Although this "speed versus accuracy" tradeoff has been known in psychology for over 100 years, it has only recent-ly been addressed in people with MS. Recent data suggest that pro-cessing speed is impaired irrespective of performance accuracy.

In two recent studies, people with *relapsing-remitting* MS demonstrated impairments in processing speed but intact working memory, whereas people with *secondary-progressive* MS showed impairments in both processing speed and working memory.[11–12] These results support the hypothesis that speed of information pro-cessing may be slowed early in the disease (when the disease is relapsing-remitting), whereas deficits in working memory become prominent with disease progression (when and if the disease becomes secondary-progressive).

It is easy to see that if a person with MS is experiencing difficul-ties in the speed with which information is processed, this could clearly affect the quality of information that he or she is able to learn. Think of listening to a lecture. The pace at which the teacher presents the material is the same for all students in the class. However, if the person with MS cannot keep up with the points that are being made, he or she will learn less information, or the quality of that information will be deficient. We know from the previous section that if information is not adequately learned, it will not be stored properly in the brain, and its recall will be less than what the teacher requires on the exam. Thus, processing speed can have pro-found consequences in everyday life.

Fortunately, some very preliminary research suggests that, given an adequate amount of time, the quality of the information processed by someone with MS can be improved to the level of the general population.[13] This research is, however, very preliminary, and further work is needed.

Executive Functions

Executive functions consist of "those capacities that enable a person to engage successfully in independent, purposive, self-serving behav-ior."[17] It represents the highest level of human cognitive processes. Executive functions include the following abilities: planning; organ-ization; initiation of tasks; problem-solving, reasoning, and concept formation; and self-awareness. Because of the wide spectrum of abil-ities associated with executive functions, the nature of an executive problem (if any) varies greatly from one individual to another.

Despite the wide spectrum of executive functions, neuropsycho-logic research has focused primarily on a narrow range of abilities, primarily abstract and conceptual reasoning and set-shifting (i.e., having the mental flexibility to shift from one concept to another when trying to solve a problem). The available research clearly shows that people with MS can experience difficulties in solving complex problems. Such difficulties in solving problems can arise from difficulties in planning, organization, and/or reasoning and conceptualization.

It is important to understand that what people with MS experience or report as memory problems may, in fact, be problems with executive functions. For example, being less organized in one's thinking could make a person less careful about leaving the car keys in the same spot everyday. Or, reduced planning abilities may result in "forgetting" to bring the grocery list to the store. Such executive problems might seem like "losing one's memory," but may actually reflect the impact of deficient executive skills on remembering.

Visual Perceptual Functions

Visual perceptual functions refer to the perception of visual information. Because we interact and learn from our world in large part through vision, how we perceive the environment greatly affects our mental development, fund of knowledge, and everyday interactions. As such, visual perceptual functions are critical, yet very complicated. Such perception includes everything from simple object recognition (ranging from simple shape and surface detail to object naming), to matching visual input with mental images already stored in the brain, to semantic categorization (e.g., matching the visual image to what it actually means). It has been suggested that up to about one-quarter of people with MS have significant difficulty with visual perceptual skills.[18]

To start with, people with MS can have difficulties in basic visual sensory functions, typically from optic neuritis (inflammation of the optic nerve), which can result in blurred vision. This faulty visual input has the potential to affect higher-level visual perception (e.g., face recognition, judging spatial distance) and affect everyday life activity (e.g., driving). In addition to primary sensory disturbances, some people with MS have been shown to experience difficulties in visual object recognition,[19] color discrimination,[18] and visual perception and visual discrimination.[20] Unfortunately, compared to learning and memory, relatively little research has examined the nature of visual perceptual problems in MS and their impact on everyday life.

Intellectual Functions

Intelligence is a broad term with multiple meanings across various groups and disciplines (e.g., anthropologists, psychologists). Clinically, it is most often measured by IQ (Intelligence Quotient), which is actually a fairly narrow representation of the broad concept of intelligence. Overall, intellectual functions are thought to be preserved in people with MS.[21-22] Although some studies show some level of decline on IQ tests among people with MS, this reduced level of performance is typically caused by the nonintellectual aspects of traditional IQ testing, such as sensory-motor impairment (e.g., from sensory changes or weakness in the hands that slow a person's ability to manipulate objects) or slowed processing speed, which affect some aspects of IQ testing more than others. For those components of IQ tests that are less sensitive to sensory-motor problems (e.g., verbal intelligence), little if any drop in IQ is observed among people with MS. Although generally preserved, however, one should recognize that a small subset of people with MS may exhibit intellectual decline, particularly those with very severe deficits.

Language Functions

Impairment in language functions in MS is relatively rare. That is, the ability to comprehend language and express oneself, as well as naming and verbal repetition, are primarily intact.[22] However, word-finding difficulties (the "tip-of-the-tongue" phenomenon) are a common problem in everyday life. Another common, and likely related, difficulty is word fluency, as in generating words from a category (e.g., listing all the words one can think of that start with the letter "C"). It is likely that both word finding and word fluency are related to reduced speed of processing or the speed of retrieving information from long-term storage.

Overall, decreased cognitive efficiency can be a significant reality for people with MS. When present, cognitive problems generally are found in the areas of reduced information-processing speed, problems in the adequate learning of new information, and difficulties in multitasking. Areas of cognition that are generally unaffected by MS are overall intellectual skills and verbal and language processing. Cognitive problems do not occur in everyone with MS and, when they do, may range from mild to moderate to severe, with mild to moderate being most likely. Although terms like mild, moderate, and severe may describe the magnitude of the cognitive problem, it is recognized that even a "mild" cognitive problem may have a "severe" impact on one's quality of life and on how a person feels about him- or herself.

HOW DO COGNITIVE PROBLEMS AFFECT THE PERSON WITH MS?

"I thought I was losing my mind. It was difficult to explain to others what was happening when I didn't know myself. I do remember the fear and loneliness that went along with all this. I silently begged God, 'Do what you will to my body, but please leave my mind alone.'"[23]

Realizing that cognitive problems are indeed a symptom of MS can be both extremely difficult to accept and live with, but also very reassuring. People are relieved to know that they are not "going crazy," or as a person with MS described it—"Look—I'm 'normally' abnormal."[23]

Impact on Quality of Life

Research has shown that cognitive dysfunction among people with MS can result in significant disruptions in daily activities, lifestyle, employment status, social functioning, as well as overall quality of life.[24,25] Although physical disability can have obvious effects on quality of life, so can the cognitive impairments associated with MS. In one study, MS participants with cognitive and physical impairments were compared to a group of MS participants with only physical impairments on measures of quality of life.[20] The two MS groups were matched for disease course (e.g., relapsing-remitting MS versus secondary-progressive MS), disease duration (time since diagnosis), and demographic variables (including age and education). The study found that cognitively impaired individuals with MS were less likely to be employed, were engaged in fewer social and vocational activities, and had greater difficulties in carrying out routine household tasks, when compared with the purely physically-impaired MS group.

Another study[26] showed that challenges in activities of daily living were related to difficulties in learning new information, which we know from the preceding discussion to be one of the key cognitive problems experienced by people with MS. Another study[27] demonstrated that the extent of cognitive impairment significantly impacts social and vocational quality of life, regardless of the degree of physical disability.

Unemployment rates in the MS population are as high as 84% for women and 72% for men—drastically higher than those observed in the normal population.[24] Both physical and cognitive impairments contribute to early retirement in as many as 80% of individuals with MS.[28-29] Yet, one study found that physical disability and demographic factors (such as age, sex, or education) have much less of an impact on employment status in MS than other factors, including cognitive symptoms.[30]

Although many factors have been shown to be related to employment status in MS, including the presence of a working spouse, age, duration and course of disease, severity of physical symptoms, fatigue, and visual impairment, individuals with MS have identified information processing and memory deficits as presenting significant obstacles to maintaining meaningful employment.[31] In fact, the unemployment rate among people with MS with no reported cognitive problems was found to be 53%, compared with 86% in people with MS who reported experiencing cognitive problems.[32] Individuals with MS who maintained employment performed significantly better on cognitive testing than those who were unemployed.[33] In this study, information processing efficiency and memory performance were the two cognitive abilities that had the greatest impact on work status.

Another study compared people with MS who had predominantly brain lesions to those with predominantly spinal cord lesions and noted that, despite their greater physical disability, the group with spinal lesions was more likely to be employed than was the group with brain lesions.[34]

Driving

The influence of cognitive factors on driving in people with MS is an area that has recently received specific attention. Given that driving is associated with social independence in our society, the loss of driving ability can have significant negative personal and social consequences. Although it is clear that the physical difficulties that are often associated with MS can present challenges to driving ability, research has shown that cognitive impairment in MS may also affect one's ability to drive. For example, recent studies have shown that impairments in information-processing speed and working memory are significantly correlated with overall performance on computerized tests designed to assess driving skills.[35] When MS participants with minimal or no physical disabilities were evaluated on a computerized driving assessment task, those with cognitive impairment performed more poorly.[36] These same participants also had higher numbers of actual motor vehicle crashes in everyday life.[37]

These research findings should not be interpreted to mean that people with MS-related cognitive problems must immediately stop driving. What they do suggest, however, is that people with MS and their families should take a long and honest look at the individual's profile of cognitive abilities, as well as his or her driving skills, and talk to the physician about whether driving should be assessed by a professional and/or modified (e.g., no driving at night, driving only in local or familiar places, etc.), or stopped altogether. Although the physician can assess the person's neurologic status, the professional driving evaluation is the best way to assess systematically one's ability to drive safely. The driving evaluation assesses both physical (ability to manipulate the pedals quickly and easily, and manipulate the steering wheel) and cognitive (ability to attend to environmental stimuli, make appropriate decisions, and react quickly) aspects of driving. Many rehabilitation hospitals offer driver evaluations. You can contact the National Multiple Sclerosis Society (1-800-FIGHT-MS; 1-800-344-4867) for information about facilities in your area that offer this service.

It is important to note that the reporting requirements for physicians vary from state to state. In some areas, doctors who determine that a person is too impaired to drive are required to report this finding to the Department of Motor Vehicles; other states have no such requirement for doctors. This means that some physicians are much more vigilant than others about their patients' driving abilities. In fact, many people with MS have altered their own driving habits despite being given the "green light" by their physician.

Self-Confidence and Self-Esteem

Overall, the literature is clear that the cognitive problems experienced by people with MS can have a significant impact on employment status, social and family functioning, and overall quality of life.

Beyond the research questionnaires and experiments that attempt to document the impact on everyday life, clinical experience reveals that cognitive dysfunction has a very personal effect on daily life. Difficulty in finding the right words, feeling as though you cannot follow a social conversation or understand a joke, being unable to remember to make the phone call that your friend is expecting from you—these are all examples of common problems that can be embarrassing and upsetting. The feeling that one is "stupid" or "can't keep up" can lead to social and family isolation, and perhaps depression and other problems (e.g., weight gain, losing one's job, decreased interest in doing what was once enjoyable, etc). For a person with MS, the key is to understand the specific nature of his or her cognitive problems and what they truly involve. People with MS do not become "less intelligent." Although one can begin to feel that way because of problems with slowed processing speed or impaired memory, for example, separating the feeling from the knowledge of the actual cognitive problem(s) is the first step in avoiding the downhill plunge into self-criticism and despair.

HOW DO COGNITIVE SYMPTOMS RELATE TO OTHER ASPECTS OF THE DISEASE?

"It happens to everybody. You're just getting older."[24]

Many misconceptions and misunderstandings exist about how cognitive problems are related to other MS symptoms. Some of these are explored in this section.

Relationship with Physical Disability

Most physicians and other health care providers believe that MS-related cognitive problems are correlated with physical disability. However, the majority of studies to date have found little to no relationship between cognitive problems and the degree of physical disability in people with MS. For example, physical disability (usually measured by the *Expanded Disability Status Scale [EDSS]*) explains only 10%–15% of the differences in neuropsychologic performance when other variables such as age or education are taken into account.[38]

Most of these studies are cross-sectional in design—meaning that they examine cognition in many individuals at a single point in time—and thus do not take into account how cognition changes over time. A few studies have taken a more longitudinal approach to address the question of how cognitive functioning changes over the course of the disease. One recent study examined cognition and physical disability over a 10-year period.[27,39] This work showed that, over the first four years of the disease, cognitive impairment and physical disability did not necessarily follow the same course.[27] A different pattern emerged, however, when the same subjects were re-examined 10 years after the initial testing. By 10 years later, physical disability (as measured by the EDSS) was significantly correlated with the degree of cognitive impairment.[27] This is discussed more fully in the next section.

Taken together, what these data reveal is that cognitive problems can occur whether one has physical symptoms or not, particularly early in the course of the disease. As the disease progresses over time, however, the physical impairment and cognitive deficits tend to converge. Thus, the chances gradually increase of having physical and cognitive problems together.

Course of the Disease

It used to be said that cognitive symptoms only appeared later in the progression of the disease. We know today that this is incorrect. Cognitive impairment can be observed at any time in the course of MS—or not at all. This means that some newly-diagnosed individuals can have cognitive changes among their earliest symptoms, although other people, diagnosed decades earlier, have no cognitive impairments.

In general, cognitive impairment is less severe in people with a relapsing-remitting (RRMS) disease course than in those with a secondary-progressive (SPMS) course.[12] For example, the relative risk of having an impairment in information-processing speed in RRMS is about five times higher than that observed in the general population. In contrast, the relative risk in SPMS jumps to 65 times that observed in the general population.[12] However, this cognitive differential may have little to do with disease course (or subtype) itself and more to do with disease progression. About 80%–90% of people with RRMS transition to SPMS within 25 years. Thus, by definition, disease duration is longer in SPMS, and the degree of neurologic disability (EDSS) is greater in SPMS than in RRMS. Furthermore, the extent of damage to brain structures is generally greater in SPMS than in RRMS.[40]

Understanding what happens to cognitive dysfunction over the course of the disease has been challenging, resulting in inconsistent findings across studies. As mentioned, the cross-sectional nature of most of these studies has made it impossible to determine what happens over the long run. For instance, one study examined two groups of MS participants—"cognitively mildly deteriorated" and "cognitively preserved." The investigators found that, after three years, those who were "cognitively mildly deteriorated" at the beginning showed progressive decline. In contrast, those who were "cognitively preserved" at the beginning remained stable three years later.[41] In general, disease duration, disease course, and level of neurologic disability were unrelated to cognitive decline. However, other studies that have looked at short spans of time have found no significant cognitive decline at one- to four-year follow-ups.[42,32]

In the longest follow-up study performed to date, individuals with MS were examined at four and again at 10 years after initial cognitive assessment.[27] The investigators found that as the disease progresses, the number of people with cognitive problems tends to increase (Table 3.2). For example, the percentage of MS participants with no cognitive impairment fell from 74% at initial testing to 51% at four-year follow-up and to 44% at the 10-year follow-up. Those with mild impairment from the beginning became more impaired by the time of the four-year follow-up and subsequently leveled off. MS participants who experienced moderate cognitive impairment initially tended to remain approximately the same or became slightly more impaired.

Fatigue

Self-reported fatigue is the most common symptom of MS, affecting about 90% of people with the disease. People with MS experience fatigue as extreme lassitude and tiredness, and a lack of energy that is out of proportion to the type of activity that one is engaged in. Despite years of complaints that feelings of fatigue can interact with cognitive impairment, only recently has research begun to address this issue.[44]

TABLE 3.2. Evolution of cognitive dysfunction in MS over a 10-year period

	Percent of group impaired		
MS grouping	Initial testing	4-Year follow-up	10-Year follow-up
No impairment	74%	51%	44%
Mild impairment	8%	33%	34%
Moderate impairment	18%	16%	22%

Adapted from Amato MP, Ponziani G, Siracusa G, Sorbi S. Cognitive dysfunction in early-onset multiple sclerosis. *Arch Neurol* 2001;58:1602–1606.

Does self-reported fatigue result in decreased cognitive performance (referred to as *cognitive fatigue*)? One of the difficulties in answering this question lies in how cognitive fatigue is defined. There are several ways to think about this. First, cognitive fatigue can be thought of as decreased performance over a prolonged period of time, such as over the course of a workday. Studies in this area have examined cognitive performance after long sessions of work activity. Collectively, such studies show little to no measurable effect of prolonged effort on actual cognitive performance. Although participants reported greater feelings of fatigue with prolonged cognitive activity, they did not, in fact, perform less well.[45–47]

Another way to think about cognitive fatigue is to compare it with how motor or muscle fatigue has been examined—that is, during sustained mental effort (maintaining constant cognitive vigilance) rather than prolonged mental effort (performing tasks over the course of a work day, but without constant or sustained effort). When required to sustain continuous mental effort on a challenging task, people with MS show a gradual deterioration in performance (e.g., from the first half to the second half of a long task).[10,48–49] These data suggest for the first time that we may be able to objectively measure cognitive fatigue in people with MS.

Levels of self-reported fatigue have generally not been related to cerebral abnormalities (e.g., total amount of lesion area in the brain or amount of brain atrophy) as measured by structural *magnetic resonance imaging (MRI)* or ratings of neurologic disability (e.g., EDSS), even when fatigued and nonfatigued subjects are compared.[50] Using *functional MRI (fMRI)* or *positron emission spectroscopy (PET)* scans, some preliminary data demonstrate a relationship between self-reported fatigue and simple motor performance that involves the frontal lobes and basal ganglia.[51–52] However, the relationship between self-reported fatigue and brain mechanisms on cognitive tasks remains unclear.

Overall, self-reported fatigue does not appear to be a good measure of the actual effects of fatigue on performance.

Depression

Although depression is a significant problem for many people with MS, and one that directly affects quality of life, the research examining the relationship between depression and cognitive impairment in people with MS has been mixed. Initial studies have found little or no correlation between cognitive impairment and depression.[6,15]

Such studies, however, have used a correlational approach that some argue is less sensitive to the impact of depression on cognition.[53] A meta-analysis (a technique used to analyze the results of several published studies at the same time) did find a significant relationship between depression and working memory performance.[54]

Other recent neuropsychologic studies have directly compared the performance of people with MS who were depressed with the performance of MS participants who were not depressed. Such studies have found that people with MS who are depressed perform more poorly on tasks that require a lot of effort (e.g., working memory, processing speed) compared with those with MS who are not depressed.[55–56] The two MS groups did not differ on tasks requiring less "effort" to complete. In another recent study, although both depressed and nondepressed people with MS were impaired in learning and memory performance when compared with people without MS, the depressed MS group did significantly worse than the nondepressed MS subjects.[53]

Such studies suggest that depression may increase the severity of cognitive problems, particularly in effortful and challenging cognitive situations. These data imply that the treatment of depression may improve cognitive performance somewhat (at least the component affected by depression). However, this specific hypothesis has not been studied yet.

Stress

The relationship between stress and MS is complex and not well understood. Although it is commonly thought that stress may affect cognitive processes in people with MS, little research specifically addresses this relationship in MS. It is generally accepted, however, that stress can affect cognition and mood in humans.[57] This effect is mediated by a variety of physiologic systems—including the *autonomic nervous system*, the *hypothalamic-pituitary-adrenal (HPA) axis*, and the *immune system*—all of which are known to be altered in MS. However, the study of the influence of stress on cognitive functioning in MS is in its infancy. One study found that overall cognitive status (assessed by a brief screening test) was associated with current psychological distress but not with distress over one's lifetime.[58] HPA hyperactivity has recently been shown to be related to increased cognitive impairment in people with MS.[59] However, any potential relationship with stress was not examined in this study.

THE COMPLEX INTERACTIONS AMONG STRESS, DEPRESSION, AND COGNITIVE FUNCTION

We all recognize that issues such as stress, depression, and cognitive impairment, although often studied in isolation, actually interact with each other and with other variables in a very complex way. Thus, in everyday life, it would be appropriate to ask how stress affects depression, which itself may influence cognitive processing and hence, everyday life. For example, does the way an individual copes with stress influence whether he or she becomes depressed? And does that, in turn, influence his or her cognitive functioning?

One group of researchers has made an initial attempt to explore this complex relationship.[60] They found that cognitively impaired individuals who used maladaptive coping strategies to deal with stress were much more likely to be depressed than those who employed effective coping mechanisms. Such data show that the use of particular coping strategies can either serve as a risk factor (when the strategies are maladaptive) or a protective mechanism (when the strategies are effective) for experiencing depression, which, in turn, can further complicate cognitive difficulties. And together, these can all affect everyday functional activities.

The work is just beginning on the influence of stress on cognitive functioning in people with MS, and there is plenty of room for influential research in the future.

WHAT IS THE IMPACT OF COGNITIVE DYSFUNCTION ON EVERYDAY LIFE?

We have learned that cognitive difficulties are a reality in one-half to two-thirds of people with MS. These cognitive impairments are a direct result of damage to neurons in the brain, including demyelination, which reduces transmission speed, and axonal damage, which can block nerve transmission altogether.[40] But, we also know that other factors can influence the experience of cognitive difficulties in everyday life, such as depression, fatigue, and stress. How does this all work together to provide the experience of impaired cognition in everyday life? Primary and secondary factors determine how cognition is affected in everyday life:

Primary factors refer to the actual effect of reduced brain efficiency on cognitive performance (i.e., the direct impact of neural damage on cognition). We know that measures of brain lesions using

MRI (e.g., total lesion load, brain atrophy, cerebral metabolism) and other techniques (electrophysiologic techniques, such as *evoked potentials*) are significantly related to cognitive impairment across a number of studies.[4] Thus, a direct or "primary" effect occurs in people with MS, and this effect is responsible for the cognitive impairments that they experience. Most research studies are documenting these primary cognitive factors in MS.

Secondary factors include variables that can change from day to day, or over periods of time—such as depression, fatigue, stress, the side effects of some medications—which can influence the experience of impaired cognition. Often, in everyday life, it is the impact of these "secondary" factors on cognitive functioning that can "feel" most debilitating. For example, the real-life experiences of not being able to find the right word during conversations, or feeling pressured to respond more quickly than one is able, can lead to loss of self-esteem and/or feelings of anxiety and embarrassment. These uncomfortable feelings act in a secondary way to further diminish a person's mental sharpness, resulting in the feeling of impaired cognitive efficiency and significantly influencing everyday life activities. It is often these very specific examples in everyday life that feel most debilitating, and that people with MS describe to their health care providers as evidence of their cognitive challenges.

Although much of the research on cognition in MS has focused on the primary factors, these secondary factors should not be ignored—especially by people with MS. It is very important for someone with MS to take a good hard look at him- or herself and try to recognize how such secondary factors might be affecting daily activities at work and at home. These factors can be treated effectively, thus improving the everyday life experience of cognitive dysfunction. If left unchecked, these secondary factors can themselves become the reasons for clinical depression, social isolation, or problems at work or home.

Thus, the actual experience of cognitive problems in everyday life is a complex interaction between the primary factors that cause cognitive difficulties (e.g., reduced processing speed, difficulties in learning and memory) and the secondary factors that further reduce what is already an inefficient processing system. The recognition of having "problems with my brain" is not enough. Stress, fatigue, lack of sleep, reduced physical fitness, medication, and a host of other life experiences can also affect one's experience of cognitive efficiency. Understanding how these factors interact at a personal level can be one of the best things that any person with MS can do to improve his or her quality of life.

36   *References*

1. Peyser JM, Rao SM, LaRocca NG, Kaplan E. Guidelines for neuropsy-chological research in multiple sclerosis. *Arch Neurol* 1990;47:94–97.
2. Rao SM. Cognitive function inpatients with multiple sclerosis: Impairment and treatment. *Int J MS Care* 2004;1:9–22.
3. Squire LR. *Memory and Brain*. New York: Oxford University Press, 1987.
4. Markowitsch HJ. Memory and amnesia. In Mesulam MM (ed.), *Principles of Behavioral and Cognitive Neurology*. New York: Oxford University Press, 2000.
5. Brown SC, Craik FIM. Encoding and retrieval of information. In Tulving E, Craik FIM (eds.), *The Oxford Handbook of Memory*. New York: Oxford University Press, 2000.
6. DeLuca J, Barbieri-Berger S, Johnson SK. The nature of memory impairment in multiple sclerosis: acquisition versus retrieval. *J Clin Exp Neuropsychol* 1994;16:183–189.
7. DeLuca J, Gaudino, EA, Diamond BJ, et al. Acquisition and storage deficits in multiple sclerosis. *J Clin Exp Neuropsychol* 1998;20: 376–390.
8. Gaudino E, Chiaravalloti N, DeLuca J, Diamond BJ. A comparison of memory performance in relapsing-remitting, primary-progressive and secondary progressive multiple sclerosis. *J Neuropsychiatr Neuropsychol Behav Neurol* 2001;14:32–44.
9. Demaree HA, Gaudino EA, DeLuca J, Ricker JH. Learning impairment is associated with recall ability in multiple sclerosis. *J Clin Exp Neuropsychol* 2000;22:865–873.
10. Bryant D, Chiaravalloti ND, DeLuca J. Objective measurement of cognitive fatigue in multiple sclerosis. *Rehab Psychol* 2004;49: 114–122.
11. Archibald CJ, Fisk JD. Information processing efficiency in patients with multiple sclerosis. *J Clin Exp Neuropsychol* 2000;22:686–701.
12. DeLuca J, Chelune GJ, Tulsky D, et al. Is processing speed or working memory the primary information processing deficit in multiple sclerosis? *J Clin Exp Neuropsychol* 2004;26(4):550–562.
13. Demaree HA, DeLuca J, Gaudino EA, Diamond BJ. Speed of information processing as a key deficit in multiple sclerosis: Implications for rehabilitation. *J Neurol Neurosurg Psychiatr* 1999;67:661–663.
14. Kail R. Speed of information processing in patients with multiple sclerosis. *J Clin Exp Neuropsychol* 1998;20:98–106.
15. Rao SM, St. Aubin-Faubert P, Leo GL. Information processing speed in patients with multiple sclerosis. *J Clin Exp Neuropsychol* 1989;11: 471–477.
16. De Sonneville LM, Boringa JB, Reuling IEW, et al. Information processing characteristics in subtypes of multiple sclerosis. *Neuropsychologia* 2002;40:1751–1765.
17. Lezak MD. *Neuropsychological Assessment*, 3rd ed. New York: Oxford University Press, 1995.

18. Vleugels L, LaFosse C, van Nunen A, et al. Visuoperceptual impairment in multiple sclerosis patients diagnosed with neuropsychological tasks. *Mult Scler* 2000;6:241–254.

19. Laatu S, Revonsuo A, Hamalainen P, et al. Visual object recognition in multiple sclerosis. *J Neurol Sci* 2001;185:77–88.

20. Rao SM, Leo GJ, Bernardin L, Unverzagt F. Cognitive dysfunction in multiple sclerosis: frequency, patterns and prediction. *Neurology* 1991;41:685–691.

21. Bobholz JA, Rao SM. Cognitive dysfunction in multiple sclerosis: a review of recent developments. *Curr Opin Neurol* 2003 16:283–288.

22. Wishart H, Sharpe D. Neuropsychological aspects of multiple sclerosis: a quantitative review. *J Clin Exp Neuropsychol* 1997;19:810–824.

23. Hall K. About...um...I forgot!! *InsideMS* 1999;17:52–53.

24. Kornblith AB, LaRocca NG, Baum HM. Employment in individuals with multiple sclerosis. *Int J Rehab Res* 1986;9:155–165.

25. LaRocca NG. *Employment and Multiple Sclerosis.* New York: National Multiple Sclerosis Society, 1995.

26. Kessler HR, Cohen RA, Lauer K, Kausch DF. The relationship between disability and memory dysfunction in multiple sclerosis. *Int J Neurosci* 1992;62:17–34.

27. Amato MP, Ponziani G, Siracusa G, Sorbi S. Cognitive dysfunction in early-onset multiple sclerosis. *Arch Neurol* 2001;58:1602–1606.

28. Gronning M, Hannisdal E, Mellgren SV. Multivariate analysis of factors associated with unemployment in people with multiple sclerosis. *J Neurol Neurosurg Psychiatr* 1990;53:388–390.

29. Mitchell JN. Multiple sclerosis and the prospects for employment. *J Soc Occup Med* 1981;31:134–138.

30. LaRocca N, Kalb R, Schneinberg L, Kendall P. Factors associated with unemployment in patients with multiple sclerosis. *J Chron Disabil* 1985;38:203–210.

31. Roessler RT, Rumrill PD Jr. The relationship of perceived worksite barriers to job mastery and job satisfaction for employed people with multiple sclerosis. *Rehabil Couns Bull* 1995;39:2–14.

32. Edgley K, Sullivan MJ, Dehoux E. A survey of multiple sclerosis, part 2: determinants of employment status. *Can J Rehab* 1991;4:127–132.

33. Beatty WM, Blanco CR, Wilbanks SL, et al. Demographic, clinical, and cognitive characteristics of multiple sclerosis patients who continue to work. *J Neurol Rehab* 1995;9:167–173.

34. Wild KV, Lezak MD, Whitman RH, Bourdette DN. Psychosocial impact of cognitive impairment in the multiple sclerosis patient. *J Clin Exp Neuropsychol* 1991;13:74.

35. Shawaryn MA, Schultheis MT, Garay E, DeLuca J. Assessing functional status: the relationship between the multiple sclerosis functional composite and driving. *Arch Phys Med Rehab* 2002;83(8):1123–1129.

36. Schultheis MT, DeLuca J, Garay E. The influence of cognitive impairment on driving performance in multiple sclerosis. *Neurology* 2001;56:1089–1094.

37. Schultheis MT, Garay E, Millis SR, DeLuca J. Motor vehicle crashes and violations among drivers with multiple sclerosis. *Arch Phys Med Rehab* 2002;83:1175–1178.

38. Fischer JS, Foley FW, Aikens JE, et al. What do we really know about cognitive dysfunction, affective disorders, and stress in multiple sclerosis? A practitioner's guide. *J Neurol Rehab* 1994;8:151–164.

39. Amato MP, Ponziani G, Pracucci G, et al. Cognitive impairment in early-onset multiple sclerosis: patterns, predictors, and impact on everyday life in a 4-year follow-up. *Arch Neurol* 1995;52:168–172.

40. Herndon RM. *Multiple Sclerosis: Immunology, Pathology, and Pathophysiology.* New York: Demos Medical Publishing, 2003.

41. Kujala P, Portin R, Ruutiainen J. The progress of cognitive decline in multiple sclerosis: a controlled 3-year follow-up. *Brain* 1997;120:289–297.

42. Hohol MJ, Guttmann CRG, Orav J, et al. Serial neuropsychological assessment and magnetic resonance imaging analysis in multiple sclerosis. *Arch Neurol* 1997;54:1018–1025.

43. Jennekins-Schinkel A, Laboyrie PM, Lanser JBK, van der Velde EA. Cognition in patients with multiple sclerosis after four years. *J Neurol Sci* 1990;99(2–3):229–247.

44. DeLuca J. Fatigue, cognition and mental effort. In DeLuca J (ed.), *Fatigue as a Window to the Brain.* Boston: MIT Press, 2005.

45. Beatty WW, Goretti B, Siracusa G, et al. Changes in neuropsychological test performance over the workday in multiple sclerosis. *Clin Neuropsychol* 2003;17:551–560.

46. Johnson SK, Lange G, DeLuca J, et al. The effects of fatigue on neuropsychological performance in patients with chronic fatigue syndrome, multiple sclerosis, and depression. *Appl Neuropsychol* 1997;4:145–153.

47. Paul RH, Beatty WW, Schneider R, et al. Cognitive and physical fatigue in multiple sclerosis: relations between self-report and objective performance. *Appl Neuropsych* 1998;5:143–148.

48. Krupp LB, Elkins LE. Fatigue and declines in cognitive functioning in multiple sclerosis. *Neurology* 2000;55:934–939.

49. Schwid SR, Tyler CM, Scheid EA, et al. Cognitive fatigue during a test requiring sustained attention: a pilot study. *Mult Scler* 2003;9:503–508.

50. van der Werf SP, Jongen PJH, Lycklama a Nijehold, GJ, et al. Fatigue in multiple sclerosis: Interrelations between fatigue complaints, cerebral MRI abnormalities and neurological disability. *J Neurol Sci* 1998;160:164–170.

51. Filippi M, Rocca MA, Colombo B, et al. Functional magnetic resonance imaging correlates of fatigue in multiple sclerosis. *NeuroImage* 2002;15:559–567.

52. Roelcke U, Kappos L, Lechner-Scott J, et al. Reduced glucose metabolism in the frontal cortex and basal ganglia of multiple sclerosis patients with fatigue: a ^{18}F-fluorodeoxyglucose positron emission tomography study. *Neurology* 1997;48:1566–1571.

53. Demaree HA, Gaudino EA, DeLuca J. The relationship between depressive symptoms and cognitive dysfunction in multiple sclerosis. *Cog Neuropsychiatr* 2003;8:161–171.
54. Thornton AE, Raz N. Memory impairment in multiple sclerosis: a quantitative review. *Neuropsychol* 1997;11:357–366.
55. Arnett PA, Higgonson CI, Voss WD, et al. Depression in multiple sclerosis: relationship to working memory capacity. *Neuropsychol* 1999;13:546–556.
56. Arnett PA, Higgonson CI, Voss WD, et al. Depressed mood in multiple sclerosis: relationship to capacity-demanding memory and attentional functioning. *Neuropsychol* 1999;13:434–446.
57. Kemeny ME. The psychobiology of stress. *Psychol Sci* 2003;12: 124–129.
58. Aikens JE, Fischer JS, Namey M, Rudick RA. A replicated prospective investigation of life stress, coping, and depressive symptoms in multiple sclerosis. *J Behav Med* 1997;20:433–445.
59. Heesen C, Gold SM, Raji A, et al. Cognitive impairment correlates with hypothalamo-pituitary-adrenal axis dysregulation in multiple sclerosis. *Psychoneuroendocrinology* 2002;27:505–517.
60. Arnett PA, Higgonson CI, Voss WD, et al. Relationship between coping, cognitive dysfunction and depression in multiple sclerosis. *Clin Neuropsychol* 2002;16:341–355.

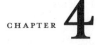

CHAPTER 4

ASSESSMENT OF

COGNITIVE CHANGES

Nicholas LaRocca, PhD, and Lauren Caruso, PhD

• •

Now that we have established that cognitive changes occur in MS, how would you know if you are experiencing these changes, and what can be done about them? The first part of this chapter describes the ways in which people are most likely to become aware of changes in their cognitive abilities. The second part talks about the benefits of addressing these changes sooner rather than later, and the remainder of the chapter outlines the steps involved in learning what you need to know about the changes you have experienced.

BECOMING AWARE OF COGNITIVE CHANGES

Cognitive changes may be noticed first by the person with MS who encounters new and unfamiliar frustrations or challenges in daily activities. Or, the changes may initially go unnoticed by the person with MS, but be picked up by family, friends, or colleagues at work.

Changes You Can Observe in Everyday Life

Cognitive changes can affect a wide variety of routine activities. In most cases, the first signs of trouble are glitches that occur in routine tasks, such as remembering appointments. Let's take a look at some of the cognitive functions that are most likely to be affected by MS and how they may play out in daily life.

MEMORY

Memory changes constitute the most common complaint in regard to cognitive functioning in MS. These are probably among the easiest to recognize because so much of everyday life involves learning, retaining, and recalling information. Here are some typical examples of ways in which memory changes might intrude on everyday activities:

- Difficulty learning and/or recalling new information
- Problems remembering the plot or characters in books
- Forgetting what was said in conversations, TV shows, movies
- Forgetting why you entered a room
- Losing or misplacing items such as glasses, keys, the TV remote
- Forgetting people's names, appointments, phone numbers
- Forgetting items on shopping trips
- Forgetting to do a task that you had planned

INFORMATION PROCESSING

Slowed information processing is another of the cognitive changes most frequently noticed in MS. Many people say that they can still do all the same things they used to be able to do, but cannot do them as quickly or efficiently as before. Examples of typical problems include:

- Productivity within a given period of time is reduced, even though the quality of the work is unchanged.
- It is difficult to respond quickly when a lot of information is presented.
- Tasks having a time element, such as card or word games or various types of work-related tasks, are more challenging.
- Processing information that is coming from several different sources at once becomes slower and more difficult.
- Planning and executing tasks becomes more difficult due to the additional time needed to complete them.

ATTENTION AND CONCENTRATION

The simple ability to "pay attention" and "concentrate" is not usually affected in MS. However, some of the more complex forms of attention and concentration are likely to be affected, causing problems like the following:

- Problems screening out distractions such as noises, thoughts, competing activities

- Difficulty with "divided attention" tasks, such as listening to what a family member is saying at the same time that you are doing something else
- Running out of steam while reading or engaging in similar tasks that require intense concentration and focus (can also involve fatigue)
- Inability to stick to one task for long without getting distracted
- Poor recall due to lack of attention when information is being learned
- Difficulties with attention that compromise your ability to organize information needed for later recall

ABILITY TO SHIFT BETWEEN TASKS

Life would be much easier if it proceeded in a straight line—if you got to finish one task before the next one required your attention. However, much of life requires that we shift back and forth between tasks. The mental flexibility that allows us to do this switching with relative ease may be affected in MS and may be compounded by slowed information processing and difficulty with attention and concentration. Examples of problems with shifting might include:

- Difficulty resuming a task after an interruption—for example, finding it hard to remember what you were doing before being interrupted by a telephone call
- Problems shifting back and forth between tasks—for example, talking with your spouse while balancing the checkbook, and then finding it difficult to remember where you are in the checkbook or what your spouse was saying to you
- Difficulty "shifting gears" when some unexpected event demands a quick but time-limited response—for example, finding it hard to turn your attention to a child's question when you are preparing dinner (described by some people as "feeling sticky")

CONCEPTUAL REASONING AND PROBLEM SOLVING

Changes in reasoning and problem solving are harder to recognize than changes in memory because reasoning involves more subtle and complex tasks than remembering where you left your keys. However, changes in conceptual reasoning and problem solving can be observed, particularly if your job or other activities involve intellectually challenging tasks. Examples might include:

- Difficulty following complex arguments or explanations
- Missing subtleties and nuances in situations, particularly complex social situations
- Trouble solving puzzles or riddles that used to be easy for you
- Slowness in understanding analogies, symbols, or metaphors
- Difficulty analyzing complex situations that formerly were easy for you
- Being too "literal" or "concrete" in your interpretation of words—such as not "getting" jokes

EXECUTIVE FUNCTIONS

What is it that "executives" do? They organize and execute complex sequences, such as running a company, a department, or a major project. We are all "executives," because life in the modern world involves many situations in which we have to organize and execute complex sequences by planning, prioritizing, sequencing, and implementing interrelated tasks. These executive functions are frequently affected in MS and can have a major impact on everyday life. Common examples of this type of problem include:

- Trouble organizing and following through with complicated tasks, such as filing income tax returns, planning a vacation, or buying a new car
- Difficulty in setting priorities, organizing time, and meeting deadlines
- Jumping from one task to another with no apparent logic
- Feeling bewildered and overwhelmed by a pending task and not knowing how or where to begin

VISUAL PERCEPTUAL FUNCTIONS AND SPATIAL ORIENTATION

People with MS may find that visual/spatial skills have been adversely affected by their MS. Examples of this type of problem include:

- Getting lost while driving, even in familiar territory (may also involve changes in memory)
- Becoming confused over right and left directions
- Having trouble assembling things (e.g., toys, furniture) from a diagram or written instructions
- Finding it difficult to understand how machines work (e.g., programming a cell phone, microwave oven, or VCR)
- Having difficulty visualizing objects from a verbal description

- Having trouble judging distances between objects (e.g., when parking a car)

OBSERVATIONS MADE BY FRIENDS AND FAMILY

Most of us don't like to admit that something about us is amiss, especially something involving mental faculties such as memory or reasoning skills. As a result, sometimes a family member, friend, co-worker, or supervisor is the first to voice concern about cognitive changes. Such concerns may get a rather frosty reception from the person with MS who is not about to admit to changes of this kind. Denial is an understandable reaction to emerging cognitive changes, but it is more likely to mask the truth from the person with MS than from concerned others. These observations by others may provide the stimulus needed to begin the process of dealing with cognitive changes.

Friends and family are not always on target, however, when they react to cognitive changes. Even people familiar with MS may be unaware that the disease can affect cognition. As a result, when a person with MS starts to forget things, family members may react with frustration, thinking that it's all due to laziness, indifference, "attitude," depression, or any number of other explanations. This frustration may, of course, be their own form of denial: No one likes to think that a loved one or close friend is experiencing a change in his or her cognitive abilities. Clarifying the why and wherefore of cognitive changes can help to relieve some of the tensions that arise due to misunderstanding these changes. Even when accurately recognized, however, cognitive changes can lead to significant family strain, especially if the person with MS is running into a lot of difficulty functioning in everyday life. In such instances, a professional assessment of the changes and supportive counseling for all may be useful in learning to live with the effects of MS on cognition.

THE BENEFITS OF ADDRESSING COGNITIVE CHANGES SOONER RATHER THAN LATER

Most people who experience cognitive changes have one of two reactions: either they want to learn as much as possible about the subject, or they want to ignore it and hope it goes away. Because cognitive symptoms are as common as some of the physical symptoms of MS, it makes sense to address them as soon as possible. Although ignoring cognitive change may initially seem easier and less anxiety provoking, learning about MS-related cognitive changes will make it possible for you to:

- Clear up uncertainty and confusion concerning what's happening to you (the relief of knowing that you are not "losing your mind")
- Understand the nature of any problems you may be experiencing
- Help friends and family to understand what is happening and why
- Take steps to address the problems as soon as possible, including assessment and treatment, particularly establishing an accurate baseline against which to compare any future changes

THE STEPS INVOLVED IN LEARNING WHAT YOU NEED TO KNOW

Several steps are involved in becoming informed about MS-related cognitive changes—some involving general information-gathering, and others more specifically related to the changes you have been experiencing.

Gathering Information

A number of valuable sources of information are available concerning MS-related cognitive changes, including the National Multiple Sclerosis Society's website (go to www.nationalmssociety.org and visit the Spotlight on cognition at www.nationalmssociety.org/spotlight-Cognition). In addition, the Society offers print materials on cognition that you can access in the Library and Literature section of the website at www.nationalmssociety.org/Brochures, or request from your chapter by calling 800-FIGHT-MS (800-344-4867). It may also be helpful to talk to other people with MS. You will find that many others have experienced the same sorts of changes that you are having, and you may find it useful to compare notes on your reactions and efforts to cope with these changes.

At some point, you will probably want to discuss the subject of cognitive changes with family members, friends, co-workers, your boss, and others. Because most of these people do not have MS, they are not likely to have the same understanding of these changes as you or others with MS might have. However, cognitive changes have an impact not only on the person with MS but also on the people around him or her. So, eventually, your family and social circle will be drawn into this issue with you.

For example, if you find that you are forgetting things, it is probably better for the people around you to understand the reason for this rather than make up their own explanation—for example, assuming that you have an attitude problem or you don't care. You can explain cognitive changes in a matter-of-fact way as one of the symptoms of MS, perhaps pointing out that the problems you experience are noticeable but not severe. You might also want to say that MS generally affects some cognitive functions while leaving others intact. People you talk to may attempt to be reassuring, saying things like "Oh everyone is absent minded from time to time. I'm always forgetting where I left my glasses." You might want to explain that, although it is normal for everyone to have occasional cognitive lapses like forgetting something, the changes that occur in MS are different from the run-of-the-mill problems that people experience in daily life. Memory lapses caused by MS tend to be more frequent and more severe than those experienced by adults without MS, who may occasionally forget something. It is important for the people around you to understand the true nature of what is going on because you may need their collaboration and support to help you adapt to these changes.

Talking to Your Doctor

Although cognitive changes can often be recognized by the person with MS or an observant friend or family member, there is no substitute for a professional assessment of these changes. Research has shown that self-reports and family reports of cognitive changes are often inaccurate. Moreover, a professional assessment can pinpoint exactly which cognitive functions are affected and to what degree, and identify those functions that have not been affected. How do you begin? The first step should probably be to share your concerns with your neurologist and discuss the possibility of getting a professional assessment. Experience has shown that neurologists tend to vary in terms of how they handle patient reports of cognitive changes. In the past, patients were often told that cognitive changes only occur late in the course of the disease or only when the MS is severe. If the person "looked good" physically, cognitive complaints were often attributed to stress or depression. The truth is that cognitive changes can occur at any time during the course of the disease; in fact, these changes can even be among the first symptoms.

When talking to your physician about cognitive changes, it is best to be as specific as possible. Don't simply say "My memory seems to be shot." Instead, be prepared to provide a number of specific examples of how memory or other functions are not working correctly. Emphasize that these difficulties represent a definite change from your previous level of functioning, and don't be sidetracked by attempts to explain away your cognitive changes as the result of depression or stress. Be on the lookout as well for the tendency on the part of some doctors to avoid dealing with your complaints about cognitive changes. Because many physicians still do not feel comfortable or confident about addressing cognition problems, they may prefer to focus exclusively on your physical symptoms. Or, they may simply not know what to do about the problems or where to refer you. If you find that your physician is not able to steer in you in the right direction, you can obtain a referral from the National Multiple Sclerosis Society by calling 1-800-FIGHT-MS.

Having taken that first step of talking to your doctor, what should you expect in terms of a professional assessment? Anyone with MS has experienced a neurologic examination in which the physician assesses neurologic functions such as strength, coordination, reflexes, vision, sensation, and the like. A full neurologic examination will include a brief "mental status" examination. This mental status examination varies from doctor to doctor and may involve just a few questions or a more extensive assessment. In general, however, the standard neurologic examination is not particularly sensitive to cognitive changes, especially if they are subtle. And, most neurologists do not have the staff or resources to conduct a more comprehensive cognitive assessment.

The briefest mental status examination may include questions such as "What is your name?" "Where are you right now?" "What day is it?" along with the assignment to remember three simple objects and to count backwards from 100 by 7s. A more extensive mental status examination may entail a longer, standardized test such as the "Mini Mental State," a classic test widely used in Alzheimer's disease. Although these techniques may be useful for picking up severe cognitive problems, they are grossly insensitive to the often very subtle difficulties that are the hallmark of MS cognitive changes. A study completed by Dr. Janis Peyser of the Medical College of Vermont showed that the brief screening methods generally used as part of the neurologic examination missed half of those patients who actually had cognitive changes.

"Mental status" type examinations are generally not appropriate in MS for three reasons. First, many of the deficits seen in MS are mild to moderate and are not detected by the typical mental status examination. Second, the typical mental status examination evaluates a very limited list of functions, and it may miss any of a wide variety of functions that can be affected by MS. The person with MS is likely to be high functioning in many abilities, but have specific deficits in others. Third, the cognitive deficits in MS don't generally follow a particular pattern, thus making it difficult to pick up deficits. An adequate assessment of cognitive changes in MS requires something more than a brief mental status or quick screening test such as the Mini Mental State. Ideally, these changes should be addressed through a formal neuropsychological evaluation.

THE NEUROPSYCHOLOGICAL EVALUATION

What Is It and Who Does It?

A neuropsychological evaluation is a series of different tests, each of which is designed to assess one or more specific cognitive changes. Neuropsychological evaluations can be short (a half hour or less) or long (6 to 8 hours of face-to-face contact plus additional time for scoring, interpretation, and preparation of a report). The set of tests is often referred to as a *battery*. Batteries of tests may be assembled from different sources by the examiner or purchased "off the shelf" in a pre-assembled package. In most cases, the results of the battery of tests are not combined into a single score. Instead, specific scores are generated for different functions such as verbal memory, visual memory, abstract reasoning, and the like.

Because the pattern of cognitive changes in MS varies from person to person, and because the individual's goals also vary, the evaluation must be comprehensive enough to cover a wide variety of functions and must be sensitive to the variations between individuals. Moreover, one purpose of the evaluation is to pinpoint strengths as well as weaknesses in cognitive functions, which can only be accomplished through a comprehensive evaluation.

Neuropsychological evaluations are generally performed by neuropsychologists. A neuropsychologist is a psychologist with a doctoral degree who has specialized training in the diagnosis and assessment of cognitive problems. A clinical psychologist may also administer neuropsychological evaluations, but clinical psychologists generally lack the specialized training needed to make the best use of these types of assessments. Assessment of cognitive changes can also be performed by speech/language pathologists and occupational therapists. Although these professionals undergo different kinds of training and utilize different tests to assess cognitive functioning, each of them can provide valuable insights into the nature and severity of cognitive changes.

Finding someone familiar with MS is very important. MS has many unique aspects that can affect cognitive function and its assessment—for example, MS fatigue, exacerbations and remissions, the array of medications that a person may be taking at any given time, and so on. Someone can be well-trained as a neuropsychologist but do an evaluation that is somewhat off the mark due to a lack of understanding of MS and its idiosyncrasies. The National Multiple Sclerosis Society can often help you to find the right person to do a neuropsychological evaluation.

Why Do an Evaluation?

Because considerable time and expense may be involved in a neuropsychological evaluation, it is not something to be undertaken lightly. What are some of the reasons why one would undertake this type of assessment? A thorough assessment can make it possible for you to:

- Establish a baseline for future comparison, or to evaluate the effects of a treatment that you are starting
- Assess cognitive strengths and weaknesses, especially before beginning cognitive and/or vocational rehabilitation
- Identify one or more treatable conditions (e.g., depression) that may be obscured by cognitive symptoms
- Address any questions that may arise concerning job performance and/or job accommodations

Sometimes, a person seeks an evaluation simply because he or she has a strong need to know and understand what is happening.

What Should I Expect?

The neuropsychological evaluation and its follow-up entail several steps. First, the neuropsychologist (or other professional) may want to meet with you first to get a clear sense of your complaints and other issues going on in your life. Either at that time or on the day of the evaluation, the neuropsychologist will probably do a detailed *intake interview*. The intake interview gathers information about your complaints—physical, emotional, social, cognitive, and so on— and details concerning your education and employment history, family, and other relevant aspects of your background. This information helps to place the results of testing in context. In conjunction with some of the test results, it also allows the neuropsychologist to estimate what your level of cognitive functioning was before it was affected by MS, and to form a general picture of your strengths and weaknesses pre- and post-diagnosis. An important part of this interview involves looking for other factors that may have affected your cognitive functions, such as a head injury, other diseases, fatigue, or medications you are taking. The interview will also probe for issues that may be affecting your ability to function—such as depression or family problems.

Once the actual testing begins, it may continue for several hours, in some cases 6 to 8 hours. Neuropsychologists familiar with MS will be sensitive to the effects of fatigue and will divide the testing into manageable sessions, perhaps spread over 2 days or more. The neuropsychologist will administer a variety of different tests depending in part on the nature of the problems that you have reported. Some of these tests will be very brief, taking just a few minutes. Some will take longer. You will probably find that some parts are very easy whereas others are quite difficult. This is because many of the tests progress from easy items to harder ones to determine where you stand along a range of abilities. It is important to keep in mind that no one is expected to get every item correct. Many of the tests are designed to continue until you have gotten a certain number of the harder items wrong. This may feel somewhat demoralizing but it is the standard way of finding the upper limits of abilities.

The tests will involve a wide variety of tasks, such as remembering lists of words, remembering strings of numbers, recalling arrangements of tokens on a grid, doing calculations, naming objects from pictures, recognizing an object from a "disassembled" picture, tracing paths through mazes, connecting numbered dots in the right order, and so on. The possibilities are almost limitless, and no two neuropsychologists are likely to administer exactly the same set of tests. Moreover, depending on the information gathered during the intake or from other sources, the neuropsychologist may decide to make some changes in the set of tests to capture specific data. It is therefore impossible to describe a set of tests that could be considered a standard battery. Instead, here is a "typical" neuropsychological evaluation used by a neuropsychologist who specializes in MS:

- A paper-and-pencil or computer-driven personality inventory to screen for depression and other mood and personality issues that may affect cognition
- A test of general intellectual ability to help in estimating ability prior to MS and to provide an overview of your current level of functioning
- One or more tests of conceptual reasoning (e.g., devising strategies to accomplish some task or goal)
- One or more tests of processing speed (e.g., doing rapid calculations or coding tasks such as the substitution of numbers for symbols)
- Several tests of attention and concentration, ranging from simple "working memory" tasks (e.g., retention of information for a few seconds) to complex tasks involving divided attention (e.g., focusing on a task while being distracted by another task)
- Verbal and visual memory tasks
  - Verbal memory tasks may involve learning and recalling lists of words and numbers and/or remembering stories.
  - Visual memory tasks may involve reproducing an arrangement of checkers on a checkerboard, recognizing figures that you had previously drawn, or drawing a figure from memory.
  - Combined verbal and visual memory in a single task (e.g., remembering faces and names) may be used to evaluate how well the brain's right and left hemispheres are working together.
- Tests of expressive language (e.g., accurately expressing ideas verbally, coming up with words rapidly)
- Tests of receptive language (e.g., accurately understanding ideas expressed verbally)
- Several tests of visuospatial ability, such as reproducing designs using colored blocks, identifying or reassembling pictures of familiar objects that have been split into several pieces
- Tests of motor function, especially eye–hand coordination (e.g., placing pegs in a board with holes)

The Follow-Up

At the end of the final testing session, you will probably be anxious to know how you did. The neuropsychologist may be able to offer a brief impression of the results. However, most neuropsychologists are wary of offering too much in the way of an off-the-cuff impression. Because of the nature and complexity of the tests used in a neuropsychological evaluation, the neuropsychologist will often have to spend several hours scoring and interpreting the tests and preparing a report to provide a complete and accurate picture of the results. Once the neuropsychologist has completed the scoring and interpretation of the tests, he or she should arrange for a feedback session with you. At your discretion, this session may include one or more family members. During the feedback session, the neuropsychologist will review with you what the testing showed in terms of strengths and weaknesses in various cognitive functions. The neuropsychologist will assist you in understanding what the results mean and in exploring their implications for your life at home and at work. In general, this should be done before the report is released to the referring doctor.

Most neuropsychologists will prepare a detailed report based on the intake interview and the test results, but they may vary in the way they share this information with you. Owing to the technical nature of the report, it is generally not considered a good idea to simply mail a copy of the report to the patient. One approach is to have the person (and a family member, if you choose) read the report in the neuropsychologist's office just before the feedback session. In this way, the neuropsychologist can explain in detail what the results mean and answer any questions.

Next Steps

Cognitive functions are not the only issues addressed in a good neuropsychological evaluation. Emotional changes, family issues, job-related problems, and other issues are generally explored as well. As a result, part of the follow-up may involve addressing some of these issues, such as recommending individual or family therapy, antidepressant medication, or job-related accommodations. All these may be discussed in the feedback sessions and additional sessions, if needed.

In most cases, the neuropsychological evaluation results from a referral by your doctor. The neuropsychologist will write a detailed report of his or her findings and forward this to your doctor. In addition to the feedback session with the neuropsychologist, your doctor may also want to discuss the results with you and may refer you to another professional for follow-up. For example, your doctor may prescribe a medication or change one that you are already taking and/or refer you to a neuropsychologist, speech/language pathologist, or occupational therapist for cognitive rehabilitation; a psychiatrist for further assessment and treatment of emotional changes; or a psychotherapist for counseling. These topics are discussed in detail in Chapter 5.

The results of an evaluation can also be used to support a person's request for on-the-job accommodations. The neuropsychologist (or other specialist) will help you identify specific accommodations that would make it possible for you to do your job more productively and effectively, and they may outline a course of action for you to follow.

Neuropsychological evaluations are sometimes performed to support an application for disability benefits. If this is the case, a copy of the report may be sent to the agency or group responsible for disability determination (e.g., a government agency or private insurer). In some instances, the neuropsychologist may be asked to complete a special form provided by the insurer or to prepare a letter that briefly summarizes the test results. This letter may be attached as a cover letter to the detailed report. The neuropsychologist may also speak directly to a qualified individual from your insurer (e.g., a psychologist or physician) to discuss the implications of your test results. Neuropsychologists tend to vary in terms of the approach they prefer to use in addressing disability claims. There is no one "right" way to approach this. Rather, it is important that you and the neuropsychologist both be comfortable with the approach to be used and provide the disability determination office with the highest-quality information.

Whatever the next steps may be, they involve a set of joint decisions involving you and the various health care professionals involved. Just a few short years ago, few options were available for follow-up beyond the feedback session. However, as we shall see in Chapter 5, much has changed for the better.

CHAPTER 5

TREATMENT OF

COGNITIVE CHANGES

Nicholas Larocca, PhD

∙∙

W e have examined the cognitive changes in multiple sclerosis (MS) from many different angles: how to recognize them, the best ways to assess them, how to talk about them with family, friends, employers, doctors, and others. We have also talked about steps that can be taken following a formal assessment. In this chapter, we take a closer look at the scientific evidence to support various approaches to the treatment of cognitive changes in MS. Our discussion of treatment is divided into three sections: disease-modifying agents, symptomatic treatments, and rehabilitation. In each section, we summarize a number of studies that have examined various approaches to the treatment of cognitive changes in MS. Where possible, full citations are provided for those who might be interested in reading about a given study in greater detail.

The literature on the treatment of MS-related cognitive changes is not extensive. Research on this subject was almost nonexistent until the mid 1990s. Since then, however, a slow but steady blossoming of interest has occurred in evaluating various approaches to the treatment of cognitive changes in MS. Similarly, the treatment of these changes in everyday practice has been quite limited, but is slowing increasing as we learn more about the ways in which MS affects cognition and how best to respond to these effects. During the late 1970s, the treatment of MS-related bladder dysfunction was relatively uncommon. Today, it is considered a standard part of the ongoing management of MS. In the next few years, we are likely to see the treatment of cognitive changes go through the same evolution and assume its rightful place as an integral component of the comprehensive care of persons with MS.

TERMINOLOGY

In this chapter, we use a number of terms that might be unfamiliar to readers.

Crossover trial

Some of the drug studies that we summarize used a "crossover" design. In this design, one group of patients initially receives the treatment, while a second group of patients, matched on a range of important characteristics, receives an identically appearing placebo. At a predetermined point in time, both groups begin a "washout period" during which they stop taking whatever they have been taking. This washout period is an essential condition for a crossover design because it guarantees that the treatment being studied has no effects that carry over into the next phase of the trial. Following the washout period, the group that first received the treatment gets the placebo, and the group that first got the placebo gets the treatment. Assignment to groups is generally random, and neither patients nor doctors know when either group has received the real treatment until the study is completed. The crossover design is generally considered to be more powerful than the simple *parallel group design*, in which the treatment and placebo are each administered to only a single group. Because patients are compared to themselves (on treatment versus on placebo), the study is more sensitive to the impact of the treatment.

Double-Blind

A double-blind design is one in which neither the patients being treated nor the investigators evaluating the patients know which treatment (active drug versus placebo) each patient is receiving. Random assignments to the groups is generally done by a statistician who retains a coded record of which patients are in which group. The code may be "broken" or revealed for one or more patients in the event of an emergency, but otherwise remains secret until the conclusion of the study. If the active treatment has dramatic benefits or side effects that are readily apparent, blinding may be compromised.

A placebo is an inactive "treatment" that looks identical to the active treatment being studied. Placebos are easiest to create for drug studies in which pills or capsules are administered by mouth or a liquid is injected. Placebo conditions are difficult to create for other types of treatments such as rehabilitation interventions, surgery, and other interventions.

The term *placebo group* is often confused with control group or comparison group. A *control group* is any group designed to serve as a comparison against which to measure the effects of the intervention being studied. Therefore, a control group may receive a placebo or, in some instances, another active treatment. Non-placebo control groups are often used when studying a new treatment for a condition for which effective treatments already exist. In other words, the treatment group receives the new drug being studied, while the control group receives a medication that is already in use for that condition. Non-placebo control or comparison groups are also used to study treatments for which it is difficult or impossible to create a true placebo, for example, rehabilitation.

Random Assignment

Once patients have been recruited for a study, they are assigned to the study groups (generally treatment versus placebo) using a procedure similar to the toss of a coin. This ensures that each patient entering the study has an equal chance of being assigned to either group. In practice, no coins are actually tossed; instead, complex procedures using sets of random numbers are used. Random assignment is extremely important as a way of controlling for bias in assignment to groups. For example, if random assignment is not used, it is possible that the investigators may, without realizing it, assign the patients with the best prospects for improvement to the active treatment group.

Statistical Significance

A study result—such as a difference between active treatment and placebo—is generally considered statistically significant if the observed difference between the groups could have occurred by chance less often than 1 time in 20 (that is, less than 5% of the time). However, depending on the nature of the study and the analysis, other levels of significance may be used that are stricter, such as 1 in

100 or less than 1% of the time. If the 5% level is used, any result that could have occurred by chance more often than 5% of the time is considered to be *nonsignificant*. However, a gray area exists that is referred to as a *trend*. The term "trend" is generally used to refer to a result that could have occurred on the basis of chance less often than 1 time in 10 (10% of the time), but more often than 1 time in 20 (5% of the time). Strictly speaking, results that are only "trends" are nonsignificant; however many investigators believe that it is useful to report such trends, because they are "near misses."

DISEASE-MODIFYING AGENTS

Disease-modifying agents (DMAs) include those treatments that are designed to alter the course of MS. Altering the course of MS has been defined in a number of different ways, including slowing or halting progression of disability, altering the frequency, severity or impact of exacerbations, and modifying various parameters measured through neuroimaging, such as total amount of MS *lesion* area or number of lesions. Several DMAs have been approved by the *U.S. Food and Drug Administration (FDA)* for use in MS. However, many others have been studied, and some of these studies have examined the impact of treatment on cognitive changes.

The rationale for the use of DMAs to treat cognitive changes in MS is fairly straightforward. If cognitive changes are caused by MS, then altering the course of MS should alter the course of these changes. The strongest evidence to support this assumption comes from the neuroimaging studies that were mentioned in Chapter 3. Several studies have found that cognitive changes are associated with the number of MS lesions in the brain, the total lesion area, and degree of *cerebral atrophy*. It is therefore logical to assume that any treatment that reduces the accumulation of new MS lesions in the brain would either slow or halt the progression of cognitive changes. In practice, however, confirming this assumption has been difficult. By and large, the major studies of MS DMAs have not had as their major goal the investigation of cognitive changes. As a result, the designs of these studies have not been optimized to examine potential benefits on cognition. However, because some of these studies have included cognitive assessments, they are worth looking at to see what they might tell us about the value of DMAs for MS-related cognitive changes.

Cyclosporine

Cyclosporine is an immune-suppressing agent that is widely used to prevent the immune system from rejecting organ transplants. It was studied in the mid 1980s as a potential treatment for MS based on its immunosuppressing action. The pivotal clinical trial of cyclosporine involved 547 patients with MS in a randomized, double-blind, placebo-controlled design. Of these, 317 were administered a test of attention and perceptual processing at entry to the study and then every three months through the 24 months of the trial.[1] The results showed no effects on the cognitive measure; however, the study itself failed to show any effects on its primary outcome measure, and cyclosporine was abandoned as a treatment for MS.

Methotrexate

Methotrexate is a medication that is used in the treatment of rheumatoid arthritis and certain types of cancer. It was the focus of a randomized, double-blind, placebo-controlled trial of 60 MS patients. A comprehensive neuropsychological battery of tests was administered to 40 of the 60 patients at baseline and at 12 and 24 months. In addition, a brief neuropsychological battery of tests was administered to 35 of the 60 every 6 weeks. The results showed that methotrexate had a significant positive effect on processing speed.[2]

Copaxone

Copaxone is one of the FDA-approved drugs for the treatment of MS. In a randomized, double-blind, placebo-controlled trial of 251 patients with *relapsing-remitting MS*, a brief neuropsychological battery of tests was administered to 248 patients. The test battery, which was administered at entry into the study (baseline) and at 12 and 24 months, included measures of verbal memory, visual memory, processing speed, sustained attention, and verbal fluency. Results showed no effects on any of the cognitive measures.[3] However, the trial was successful in terms of its primary outcome, and Copaxone was ultimately approved for the treatment of MS by the FDA in 1996.

Betaseron (Betaferon in Europe)

Betaseron, the first of the beta-interferons approved by the FDA for the treatment of MS, has been available in the United States since

1993. At least three studies have examined the effects of Betaseron on cognitive changes. The study that led to FDA approval in the United States. was a randomized, double-blind, placebo-controlled trial of 372 patients with relapsing-remitting MS. A small study of cognitive changes was conducted with 30 of these 372 patients. A brief neuropsychological battery of tests was administered at 24 and 48 months following entry to the study. These tests were not, however, administered on entry to the study. The battery consisted of tests of verbal and visual memory, processing speed, and mental flexibility. The results showed a significant positive effect on visual memory, specifically the ability to reproduce a picture from memory.[4]

A small study of relapsing-remitting MS compared 23 patients who were taking Betaseron to 23 controls on no treatment. This study was a nonrandomized, open-label trial in which both patients and doctors knew who was receiving treatment and who was not. A brief neuropsychological battery of tests was administered at baseline and after 12 months. The tests included measures of verbal memory, visual memory, complex attention, concentration, and verbal fluency. Of the 23 patients on Betaseron, 18 completed the study. The patients on Betaseron showed significant improvement on complex attention, concentration, and visual memory, and were stable on all other measures. The control group deteriorated significantly in complex attention, verbal fluency, and visual memory.[5]

Cognitive changes were studied in a randomized, double-blind, placebo-controlled trial of 476 patients with *secondary-progressive MS*. In this study, 236 received Betaseron and 240 received placebo. The investigators also tested 193 healthy controls. A brief battery of neuropsychological tests was administered at baseline and at 12, 24, and 36 months. The battery of tests included measures of verbal and visual memory, processing speed, and verbal fluency. A direct comparison of the treated and placebo groups showed no differences on any of the measures. However, when the two groups were compared with the healthy controls at baseline and 36 months, the placebo group was more likely to show cognitive impairment.[6]

Avonex

Avonex is one of the beta-interferons approved by the FDA for the treatment of MS, and it has been available in the United States since 1996. The most convincing evidence for the value of MS DMAs in treating cognitive changes comes from a large study of Avonex. In that study, cognitive changes were examined in 166 out of 301 patients with relapsing-remitting MS enrolled in a randomized, double-blind, placebo-controlled trial. Two neuropsychological test batteries were used. A comprehensive battery (similar to the type of clinical battery described in Chapter 4) was administered at baseline and at 24 months. In addition, a brief battery of tests was administered at baseline and every six months until 24 months. To facilitate analysis, the tests in the comprehensive battery were grouped into three composite scores, and the tests on the brief battery were combined into a single composite score. For the comprehensive battery, results showed significant positive effects of Avonex for the memory/information processing composite, a favorable but nonsignificant trend for the executive function/visual-spatial composite, and no significant effect for the verbal abilities/attention span composite. In regard to the brief battery, results showed a significant positive effect for the composite score.[7]

The Bottom Line

Evidence for the benefit of DMAs on MS cognitive changes has been modestly positive. However, many questions remain unanswered owing to the variability and mixed quality of the studies completed thus far. None of the larger studies was designed primarily to study the impact of the treatment on cognition. As a result, most of the patients enrolled did not have cognitive changes to begin with. In most cases, a very limited set of cognitive measures was used. Because of the variability in MS-related cognitive changes, using a limited set of tests runs the risk of missing important changes. The studies reported to date used a variety of different types of patients, designs, measures, and procedures, making comparisons between them very difficult. However, it is encouraging to note that the study that featured the best design and the most comprehensive measures[7] produced the strongest evidence to date for the value of DMAs in addressing cognitive changes. Once again, one can appeal to logic when evidence is in short supply and speculate that, if current and future DMAs are able to slow or halt the progression of MS, particularly its effects on the brain, then these treatments should have positive benefits on cognitive functioning over time.

SYMPTOMATIC TREATMENTS

Symptomatic treatments include those approaches that are designed to improve symptoms without altering the course of the disease. For example an antispasticity drug is used to improve the spasticity caused by MS, although such a drug would not address the underlying cause of the problem—that is, MS lesions in certain parts of the central nervous system. Most of the symptomatic treatments that we discuss are medications of various types. Although rehabilitation might also be considered a symptomatic treatment, we discuss rehabilitation in the next section.

Potassium Channel Blockers

Interest in potassium channel blockers for treating MS goes back over 20 years. These agents are thought to have potential usefulness in MS because they speed the conduction of nerve impulses in partially demyelinated nerve fibers. Several studies have examined the safety and efficacy of these agents in MS for the treatment of weakness, visual deficits, and cognitive changes, among others. One such study examined the effects of 3,4 diaminopyridine in a randomized, placebo-controlled, crossover trial of 36 patients with definite MS. This crossover study lasted 90 days, with a 30-day treatment phase followed by a 30-day washout period and then another 30-day treatment phase. Cognitive assessment included measures of verbal memory, visual memory, and working memory, administered at baseline and at 30, 60, and 90 days. Results showed no significant effects on any of the measures.[8]

The most extensively studied of the potassium channel blockers has been 4-aminopyridine (4-AP). In a four-week, randomized, placebo-controlled, crossover trial, the effects of 4-AP on cognitive functions were studied in 20 patients with definite MS. Unlike most crossover trials, this study did not use a washout period. Instead, patients were randomized to receive either 4-AP for two weeks followed by placebo for two weeks, or placebo for two weeks followed by 4-AP for two weeks. Cognitive tests included measures of verbal memory, visual memory, processing speed, and verbal fluency. Assessments were done at baseline, two weeks, and four weeks. The results showed no significant effects, but nonsignificant trends were noted in favor of processing speed and verbal memory.[9]

4-AP was also studied in a randomized, double-blind, placebo-controlled crossover trial of 62 MS patients, of whom 49 completed the study. Patients received either 4-AP or placebo for six months and then the opposite treatment for an additional six months. A comprehensive neuropsychological battery was administered, including measures of attention, working memory, verbal memory, verbal fluency, visual-spatial orientation, and abstract reasoning. Results showed no significant effects.[10]

Antifatigue Agents

Because fatigue is thought to be associated with, or to aggravate, cognitive deficits in MS, there has been interest in evaluating the effects of antifatigue agents on cognitive changes. Amantadine, a common treatment for MS fatigue, was studied in a randomized, double-blind, placebo-controlled crossover trial with 29 MS patients. Cognitive measures included eye–hand coordination, coding, verbal fluency, working memory, and complex attention. A significant improvement while on amantadine was noted only for complex attention.[11]

In a similar study, 24 patients with clinically definite MS and fatigue were studied in a randomized, double-blind, placebo-controlled crossover trial. Outcomes used in this study were not, strictly speaking, cognitive measures, but included related parameters such as reaction time and evoked potentials. No differences for reaction time were noted, but the evoked potentials were better in the amantadine group, indicating that the treatment enhanced cerebral processing speed.[12]

In a comparative study, investigators administered either amantadine, pemoline (another drug much used in the past to treat MS fatigue), or placebo to 45 MS patients in a randomized, double-blind, placebo-controlled trial. Neuropsychological tests were administered at baseline and after six weeks and included measures of working memory, verbal memory, visual memory, motor speed, and sustained attention. Results showed that patients in all three groups improved on tests of attention, verbal memory, and motor speed. However, no differences were noted among the amantadine, pemoline, or placebo groups.[13] (Note: Pemoline [Cylert] has recently been removed from the market by the FDA.)

Modafinil, also known as Provigil, has recently generated interest as a treatment for MS fatigue. Provigil was approved by the FDA for the treatment of narcolepsy, a sleep disorder unrelated to MS. However, it has also proven to be effective against MS-related fatigue.[14] A subsequent study examined whether Provigil was effective in treating attention impairment in patients taking interferon beta-1a (Avonex). Patients taking Avonex who had attention impairments were randomized to receive Provigil in addition to their Avonex, or no additional treatment. Patients were followed for two months and were evaluated using a comprehensive battery of tests that included cognitive functions, fatigue, sleepiness, and quality of life. An interim analysis with the first 22 patients to complete the study indicated that patients taking Provigil demonstrated better performance on complex attention, speed of visuomotor construction, and memory. Patients on Provigil also showed improvement on emotional well-being and mental health.[15]

Anticholinesterase Inhibitors

Acetylcholine is a neurotransmitter (a chemical that allows nerve transmissions between cells) that is thought to play an important role in memory. An enzyme known as anticholinesterase breaks down acetylcholine, thereby reducing supplies of this neurotransmitter in the brain. It has been theorized that, when supplies of acetylcholine are reduced, memory deficits occur. To counter the effects of anticholinesterase, scientists developed anticholinesterase inhibitors that limit the breakdown of acetylcholine and thereby improve memory. Such drugs have been used with some success for several years to treat the memory deficits in Alzheimer disease and other conditions.

Although MS has very little in common with Alzheimer disease, investigators in the 1980s thought it would be worthwhile to determine if anticholinesterase inhibitors might improve memory in persons with MS. The first such study administered an anticholinesterase inhibitor called physostigmine to four MS patients who had memory deficits. The double-blind, placebo-controlled, crossover study lasted six weeks, during which time patients were administered the drug for three weeks and a placebo for three weeks. During those periods when patients were receiving physostigmine, their memory for word lists was improved when compared with the placebo periods.[16] Although the results of this study were promising, the implications were limited given the small sample and the fact that the drug was administered intravenously (through a needle inserted in a vein), an impractical method for ongoing treatment.

A subsequent study of physostigmine used a form that could be taken by mouth. This study lasted eight weeks and was also a double-blind, placebo-controlled, crossover trial. The investigators examined several cognitive functions in addition to memory. They found that, although memory for lists of words improved during the periods when the drug was being taken, some other functions actually became worse.[17]

The mixed results with physostigmine encouraged researchers to examine alternatives, the most promising of which was donepezil hydrochloride, also known by its brand name, Aricept. Aricept had been approved by the FDA for the treatment of memory disorders in people with Alzheimer's disease. Like physostigmine, Aricept is an anticholinesterase inhibitor, but is taken by mouth.

An early study of Aricept was conducted in a long-term care facility with 17 MS patients who had cognitive impairment. This study lasted 12 weeks and used an open-label design in which no placebo was used and both patients and physicians knew what treatment was being administered. The investigators observed improvement on a number of functions including verbal memory, verbal fluency, visual perception, and abstract reasoning.[18] However, the results of this study must be interpreted with caution, because no blinding and no comparison to a placebo was used.

Two studies of Aricept have been completed at Stony Brook University in New York. In the first, eight MS patients were studied for six weeks. Four of the eight received Aricept and four received no treatment. As in the earlier study of Aricept, this was an open-label design with no placebo. Outcome measures included verbal and visual memory, and verbal fluency. Although no statistically significant effects were observed, nonsignificant trends in a larger study suggested that memory for word lists might be improved by Aricept.[19]

The group at Stony Brook completed a much larger study using 69 MS patients with verbal memory impairment. In a double-blind, placebo-controlled trial that lasted 24 weeks, 35 patients received Aricept and 34 received a placebo. Outcome measures included not only cognitive tests, but also patient's perceptions of treatment response and physician's perception of treatment response. Compared to those taking placebo, the patients who received Aricept showed significant improvement on all three outcome measures.[20] A larger multicenter trial is currently in progress to further evaluate the safety and efficacy of Aricept in treating MS memory deficits.

Corticosteroids

Corticosteroids have long been used to treat MS exacerbations, but few studies have examined the effect of this treatment on cognition. One such study examined 12 patients with relapsing-remitting MS who were experiencing a relapse and 12 healthy controls. Methylprednisolone was administered in divided doses over a one-week period. Outcome measures included verbal memory, working memory, verbal fluency, and abstract reasoning, administered at baseline, at the end of the one week of treatment, and two months following entry to the study. Treatment with steroids was associated with a significant negative effect on verbal memory, but this negative effect resolved within two months. No positive effects were observed.[21]

A later study examined 27 patients with relapsing MS who were receiving corticosteroid treatment for an exacerbation and 10 patients with relapsing MS who were not in an exacerbation and who were not receiving corticosteroid treatment. This was an open-label trial in which both patients and physicians knew which patients were receiving treatment and which were not. The treatment consisted of intravenous methylprednisolone for five days followed by oral methylprednisolone for 14 days. Outcome measures included the *Expanded Disability Status Scale (EDSS)*, which measures global neurologic impairment and the MS Functional Composite, which measures walking, hand function, and speed of information processing. Assessments were made at baseline and at days 5 and 20. No significant effects were observed on the EDSS, but the MSFC improved for the treated but not the untreated group.[22]

Other Treatments

Researchers have examined a number of other symptomatic treatments for MS-related cognitive changes. In one such study, pulsating magnetic fields were applied to the brains of 30 patients with MS. In this double-blind, placebo-controlled trial, 15 patients received the real treatment and 15 received sham treatment using the same equipment and procedures but without any actual magnetic fields. Unfortunately, this study did not use objective cognitive tests; it obtained patient self-report of several functions including cognition, bladder, fatigue, hand function, mobility, sensation, spasticity, and vision. A composite measure was constructed that combined all of these measures. The composite was improved in the treated group compared to the placebo group.[23] However, the cognition measure was not significant. Although this was an interesting and innovative study, the exclusive use of self-report measures rendered the results of limited interest.

Cooling has long been a popular strategy for heat-sensitive MS patients. One study examined the effects of cooling on cognitive function. Eight heat-sensitive MS patients and eight healthy controls were given two hours of cooling and two hours of sham cooling on different days. The outcome measure was a comprehensive battery of cognitive tests administered at entry to the study and after two hours of cooling or sham cooling. Although no positive effects were observed, some negative effects were noted on visual memory in both MS patients and healthy controls.[24]

Considerable interest has arisen in recent years in the use of *Ginkgo biloba* as a treatment for cognitive deficits in a variety of disorders. In a six-month randomized, double-blind, placebo-controlled trial, investigators examined the effects of *Ginkgo biloba* on 23 patients with MS. Outcome measures included a variety of cognitive tests. Positive effects were reported on attention and memory.[25]

A study of 29 MS patients examined the impact of a skin patch containing a proprietary combination of histamine diphosphate and caffeine citrate known as Prokarin. This randomized, double-blind, placebo-controlled trial lasted for 12 weeks. Twenty-two patients wore two eight-hour Prokarin patches per day while seven wore identical-appearing placebo patches for the same period. Outcome measures included assessments of fatigue, walking, hand function, and cognition. No significant difference was noted between the treatment and placebo groups in cognitive function.[26]

The Bottom Line

Thus far, the search for a definitive "memory pill" for MS has eluded us. A wide variety of symptomatic treatments have been investigated, and most have been found to be of little value. To date, the most promising approaches have involved antifatigue agents and the anticholinesterase inhibitors. One would like to see these two types of agents studied in both comparative and combination trials to determine if one is superior to the other and if they work better in tandem. As mentioned in reference to the disease-modifying agents, study design has hampered understanding of the effects of the symptomatic agents. The use of small sample sizes, limited test batteries, and differing outcome measures from study to study renders this body of evidence limited at best. We hope that the future will bring about larger and better-designed studies with more consistency between them. However, some encouraging, if tentative, results at least suggest that symptomatic treatment of MS-related cognitive deficits may some day be considered a routine part of treatment.

REHABILITATION

The third and final approach to treatment to be discussed is ***cognitive rehabilitation***, often referred to as *cognitive remediation*.

Cognitive rehabilitation has long been a prominent component of the treatment of traumatic brain injury and stroke. However, its application in MS has lagged behind these other disorders, in part due to the perception of MS as a progressive disorder. Indeed, physical rehabilitation took a long time to gain acceptance in MS because of this same bias against attempting to "rehabilitate" patients who might get worse. Although this reluctance to work with progressive conditions has not entirely disappeared from the rehabilitation field, it has diminished to a sufficient degree that physical rehabilitation and, to a lesser extent, cognitive rehabilitation, have become accepted in MS.

Restorative versus Compensatory Rehabilitation

Cognitive rehabilitation can be conveniently divided into two approaches: restorative and compensatory. The *restorative approach* attempts to improve impaired abilities such as memory or attention through the use of various types of exercises or practice drills. The underlying assumption of the restorative approach is that the brain can partially recover from injury if the individual is subjected to a carefully designed program of graded practice in the impaired functions. For example, memory deficits might be addressed through a program of computer-mediated practice in memorizing word lists of increasing length and complexity.

A term often used in the context of this approach is the *plasticity* of the brain, which suggests that the brain can partially recover lost function by rerouting damaged pathways in the brain or transferring abilities from impaired areas of the brain to intact areas. Although brain plasticity is a very appealing and hopeful concept, it is not that easy to demonstrate. Restorative treatments such as exercises and drills tend to retrain very narrowly focused skills, such as the memorization of word lists, which may have limited usefulness in actual everyday activities.

In contrast to the restorative approach, the *compensatory approach* does not attempt to improve impaired abilities, but rather to improve everyday functions through the use of strategies that "work around" the impaired abilities. As such, the compensatory approach primarily involves substitution, in which a new way of approaching a function is substituted for the old way that no longer works. For example, the restorative approach to memory deficits might involve practice in memorizing lists of words. In contrast, the compensatory approach to memory deficits might involve teaching the individual how to use a notebook to keep track of items that are likely to be forgotten.

The compensatory approach is based on the assumption that you do not necessarily need to improve an underlying ability that has become impaired to improve the function based on that ability. This same compensatory approach is used for impaired physical functions; if someone is unable to walk (impaired ability) due to weakness caused by MS, it is possible to compensate for this impaired ability by using a motorized scooter to improve the function of mobility. The key here, of course, is substitution.

In practice, the distinction between restorative and compensatory approaches is not always perfectly clear, and some overlap occurs between the two. For example, someone working with memory exercises may learn to memorize increasingly challenging word lists—in part through repeated practice, but also through some internal compensatory strategy such as grouping them into categories or associating each word with a familiar room in the house. Cognitive rehabilitation generally involves both restorative and compensatory approaches, although the compensatory type has generated the greatest interest and, to date, seems to have been the most useful.

Research Findings

Although the studies of rehabilitation interventions do not always fall neatly into groups, we have divided this discussion of research findings into those primarily related to compensatory approaches and those primarily involving restorative approaches.

COMPENSATORY APPROACHES

One of the first articles to address cognitive rehabilitation in MS did not actually report a study or present any data. Instead, it proposed an approach to cognitive rehabilitation that emphasized compensatory strategies focused on structuring, scheduling, and recording as substitutes for impaired abilities.[27]

An early published study of cognitive rehabilitation in MS involved 40 hospitalized MS patients. Half the patients were assigned to a group-based cognitive rehabilitation program that included both restorative and compensatory approaches along with psychotherapy. The other half of the group was assigned to an unstructured discussion group. Both groups met for 60 to 90 minutes three times per week. The total treatment time averaged a little over 17 hours per person. Outcome measures included a cognitive and emotional assessment battery administered at baseline, right after treatment ended and six months after the end of treatment. Immediately following treatment, significant improvement was observed in the cognitive rehabilitation group compared with the unstructured discussion group, but only in regard to depression. However, 6 months after the end of treatment, the rehabilitation group showed improved visual memory and depression, whereas the unstructured discussion group reported being more depressed.[28]

In another study that used a group approach to cognitive rehabilitation, 12 MS patients completed 24 weeks of comprehensive, three-hour-per-week sessions that focused both on cognitive symptoms and emotions. Interventions included group therapy, art and music therapy, self-regulation, visualization, guided imagery, and meditation, as well as mental and physical exercises. The control group consisted of 10 MS patients who were assigned to a 24-week waiting list (and subsequently received the identical intensive treatment following the 24-week period). Outcome measures included verbal memory, conceptual reasoning, vocabulary, information-processing speed, depression, tactile sensitivity of the hands, grip strength, and visual acuity. Compared to the waiting-list control group, the treated group showed positive effects on verbal memory, conceptual reasoning, depression, grip strength, and tactile sensitivity of the hands.[29]

A third study using a group-based approach targeted MS-related memory problems. Patients were assigned to one of two groups. One group received a single one-hour session. The other group received six one-hour sessions. The format was lecture and discussion with a handout. In both groups, participants were trained in strategies designed to improve memory over short periods of time, such as one would encounter in everyday activities. Outcome measures included a memory test and an evaluation of simulated everyday activities that require memory. Improvement was modest and about equal in both groups.[30]

A number of compensatory strategies have been developed to enhance one's ability to remember, some of which were used in antiquity. For example, the *loci strategy* was used by orators in the ancient world to help them remember parts of their speeches. In this technique, items that one needs to remember are associated with a list of familiar locations, such as the rooms in one's house. Very little research in MS has looked at these types of strategies. One study evaluated the use of the Story Memory Technique to enhance learning and recall in MS. The *Story Memory Technique* facilitates the learning, retention, and retrieval of information by weaving the items to be remembered into a simple story narrative. Twenty-eight MS patients with memory impairment were randomized either to training in the use of the Story Memory Technique or to a similar-appearing strategy that lacked the essential ingredients of the real treatment. Eight sessions were held for both strategies. Outcome measures included several different forms of verbal memory along with an evaluation of simulated everyday activities that require memory. Compared to the control group, patients in the treatment group showed improvement in their ability to memorize a list of words and in their overall assessment of treatment.[31]

Another study looked at two compensatory strategies designed to improve learning and recall—the *ridiculously imaged story technique* (RIS) and the *face–name technique* (FNT). The RIS teaches patients to embed a list of words in a humorous story containing a lot of imagery. The FNT teaches people to associate a person's name with a distinctive feature of the person's face. In this study, eight MS patients were trained in these two techniques during the course of 15 30-minute sessions two to three times per week. Outcome measures included recall of a list of 20 words, recall of 10 persons' names, a self-report of memory problems, and depression. Results showed improvement in depression but no effect on memory.[32]

The studies cited thus far have primarily emphasized the compensatory approach to cognitive rehabilitation. However, cognitive problems do not always exist in isolation. Cognitive and behavioral changes often go together. One study specifically addressed this issue. Fifteen patients with progressive MS and marked cognitive and behavioral problems were randomized to one of two conditions. Eight patients received neuropsychological compensatory training. This training was designed to enhance patient and caregiver understanding of cognitive and behavioral changes and to improve adaptation to these problems. Seven patients were assigned to a control group consisting of nonspecific supportive therapy. In both cases, 12 weekly, one-hour sessions were held with the patient and the caregiver. Outcome measures included a comprehensive evaluation of both cognitive and behavioral functions. Compared to patients in the control group, those in the compensatory training group improved on one aspect of social behavior—egocentric (overly-personalized) speech. No other differences were noted.[33]

In clinical practice, it is common to combine the restorative and compensatory approaches and to address behavioral changes as well. One study administered such a comprehensive program to 14

MS patients with cognitive impairment. The treatment consisted of twice weekly 90-minute cognitive remediation sessions and a weekly 50-minute stress management session. Cognitive remediation combined computer-assisted memory and attention training, various remedial exercises, and training in a wide variety of compensatory strategies. Although no control group was used in this study, all participants were followed for eight weeks prior to the start of treatment, to establish a baseline of functioning. The treatment period lasted 17 weeks. Outcome measures, administered at the start of the eight-week waiting period, prior to the start of treatment, and after treatment was completed, included assessment of verbal and visual memory, attention and concentration, reading comprehension, and affect (mood). No statistically significant effects were observed in any of the measures for the group as a whole. Examination of the scores for each individual indicated that there had been improvement in many cases, but that the functions that improved differed from person to person.[34,35]

RESTORATIVE APPROACHES

Restorative approaches to cognitive rehabilitation have also seen their share of research in MS, mainly focused on attention and/or memory deficits.

One of the first such studies examined attention training in 22 MS patients showing a variety of types of attention deficits. Patients were tested three times prior to the start of treatment to establish a baseline and to determine which attention functions were most in need of treatment. Each patient then received computer-mediated attention training in his or her two most impaired attention functions, once per week over a 12-week period. Outcome measures included computerized assessments of the different forms of attention along with a self-report inventory of everyday functioning. Results showed significant improvement in attention measures that persisted through a nine-week follow-up evaluation. In addition, the self-report of everyday functioning indicated fewer attention-related problems in everyday activities.[36]

The combination of attention and memory training was examined in a study of 60 MS patients who had both attention and memory deficits. Patients were randomized to one of three conditions: eight weeks of computer-assisted memory retraining, eight weeks of computer-assisted attention retraining, or no treatment. Outcome measures included 11 tests of attention and memory. The memory retraining group improved on 7 of the 11 measures, the attention retraining group improved on one measure, and the no-treatment group showed no improvement.[37]

Attention and memory retraining were also examined in a subsequent study of 82 MS patients with mild to moderate impairments in attention and memory. Half of the patients were randomized to receive computer-assisted attention and memory training, while the other half were randomized to receive training in constructional and visual-motor coordination to serve as a control group. Two sessions were held per week for eight weeks under both conditions. Outcome measures included a brief battery of cognitive, depression, and quality of life tests. Compared to the control group, the treatment group showed improvement in only one function, verbal fluency (the ability to rapidly generate words).[38]

Understanding MS–Related Memory Impairment

Some research has specifically focused on identifying the mechanisms involved in the memory problems that are so common in MS. Although it has generally been accepted that retrieval of stored memories is at the heart of these problems, some investigators have questioned whether MS patients might have a problem in the initial storage of information. This controversy has important implications for rehabilitation, because treatment would utilize different approaches, depending on the nature of the memory deficit in MS.

One study that addressed this issue evaluated whether MS patients who required more repetitions of a word list to memorize the list would do better when called upon to recall the list at a later time. The study included 64 MS patients and 20 healthy controls. All subjects were required to memorize a list of ten words. The list was repeated until a perfect score was achieved with a maximum of 15 repetitions. The expectation was that patients who needed more repetitions to memorize the list would recall it better when tested at a later time. The outcome measure was recall of the list 30 minutes, 90 minutes, and one week after the training. Contrary to predictions, patients who needed more repetitions to memorize the list recalled fewer of the words when tested later. In contrast, healthy controls who needed more repetitions to memorize the list did just as well as controls needing fewer repetitions.[39] The authors concluded that simple repetition alone is probably not an effective strategy to maximize the encoding of new information and that a more complex approach to cognitive rehabilitation is needed.

In keeping with their conclusions, this same group of investigators completed a subsequent study of 29 MS patients with verbal memory deficits for new learning. Fifteen patients were randomly assigned to the treatment group, in which they were taught the Story Memory Technique and how to use imagery and context to learn new information. Fourteen patients were assigned to the control group, in which they read stories and then had to recall as much of the story as possible as well as answer questions about the story. Eight sessions were held under both conditions. Outcome measures included a test of ability to memorize and recall a list of words and self-report of memory. Compared to controls, patients in the experimental group with moderate to severe deficits showed a significant improvement in learning, while those with mild to moderate deficits did not. Self-reported improvement was significantly greater for the patients in the experimental group regardless of the severity of their deficits.[40]

Other Studies

One of the largest studies of cognitive rehabilitation in MS randomly assigned 240 MS patients to one of three groups—a detailed neuropsychological assessment and cognitive rehabilitation, a detailed neuropsychological assessment only, or no treatment. Outcome measures included mood, activities of daily living, quality of life, and self-report of executive functions and memory. Results showed no effects on any of the outcome measures.[41]

Some studies, while not actually testing rehabilitation programs, have examined specific aspects of cognitive function in MS, and have produced important implications for rehabilitation.

One such study evaluated whether accuracy in a task was adversely affected by impaired speed of information processing, and if accuracy could be improved if more time was allowed to complete the task. Speed of information processing was evaluated in 81 MS patients and 36 normal healthy controls. An auditory task was administered to 55 patients and 16 controls, while a visual task was administered to 26 patients and 20 controls. When given more time, MS patients performed both tasks as accurately as controls. The authors suggested that MS cognitive rehabilitation should focus in part on providing additional time to strengthen the encoding of information.[42]

Another nontreatment study with implications for cognitive rehabilitation examined the concept of *strategic application abilities* (SAAs) in MS patients. SAAs involve one's ability to utilize an appropriate strategy when confronted with an unfamiliar task. In this study, the SAAs of 76 MS patients were compared to normative values; that is, the scores achieved by normal healthy controls in data collected separately and prior to the study. Measures included a test to evaluate SAA along with assessment of cognition, depression, fatigue, and everyday activities. More than three-quarters of the MS patients had some impairment of SAAs, and this impairment was not related to depression, fatigue, neurological impairment, or everyday activities. The authors concluded that SAAs should be addressed as part of cognitive rehabilitation to help patients improve their ability to cope with novel situations.[43]

Yoga is one form of treatment not easily classified as restorative or compensatory vis-à-vis cognitive dysfunction. Sixty-nine MS patients were randomly assigned either to weekly yoga classes (22), weekly exercise classes (15), or to a waiting list control group (20) for six months. Outcome measures included a comprehensive neuropsychological battery of tests, and measures of mood, fatigue, and quality of life, all administered at baseline and at the end of the six months of treatment. Compared to the waiting-list control group, patients in both the yoga and exercise groups improved in fatigue. No other effects of treatment were noted.[44]

The Bottom Line

The body of research on cognitive rehabilitation in MS presents a bewildering array of study designs, treatment approaches, outcome measures, and conclusions. In addition, the small sample sizes and short or no post-treatment follow-up periods used in many of the studies render the conclusions tentative at best. Progress in this area has been slow, and it is not likely to accelerate unless larger sample sizes, more robust designs, and consistency in outcome measures across studies are realized.

In spite of the limitations in the research, some conclusions are possible. Tentative evidence suggests the usefulness of both the restorative and the compensatory approach in MS, although it would appear that the compensatory approach has a slight edge. The restorative approaches are particularly hampered by their tendency to produce what are known as *process-specific effects*. This means that the restorative approaches tend to be good at showing improvements in the very narrowly focused outcome measures chosen to evaluate their effects, but may have limited or no carryover to everyday activities. Given the state of the research at this point, a rehabilitation approach that combines both restorative and compensatory strategies remains appropriate. However, investigators must do a better job of determining if their treatments actually help people in their daily activities and how long these effects last.

Another interesting observation is the frequency with which mood has benefited from comprehensive cognitive rehabilitation approaches in MS. This finding suggests that mood, especially depression, must be addressed in any study of cognitive rehabilitation in MS and may be the factor that benefits most from treatment. Moreover, improvements in mood may have positive effects for cognitive functioning. Cognitive changes do not happen in a vacuum and cannot be addressed without considering the individual's emotions, and family and social life. We can hope that future studies will pay closer attention to these issues and to other critical aspects of life impacted by cognitive changes, such as work.

CONCLUSIONS

Cognitive dysfunction is common and commonly misunderstood in MS. Long overlooked or denied, cognitive changes have only recently become the subject of treatment using drugs and or rehabilitation. Tentative evidence suggests that some disease-modifying agents, some symptomatic treatments, and some approaches to rehabilitation can positively impact MS-related cognitive changes. Although much has been learned thus far, much more needs to be learned before we can outline a definitive approach to the treatment of these changes. However, it is not unreasonable to think that the day will soon arrive when the treatment of MS-related cognitive deficits will be a standard part of the management of MS and will consist of a three-way attack on the problem, including disease-modifiers, symptomatic drug treatment, and cognitive rehabilitation. Research completed to date has pointed us in the right direction; now we must continue down this road to find the answers that will help persons with MS deal most effectively with cognitive changes.

References

1. Multiple Sclerosis Study Group. Efficacy and toxicity of cyclosporine in chronic progressive multiple sclerosis: a randomized, double-blinded, placebo-controlled trial. *Ann Neurol* 1990;27:591–605.
2. Goodkin DE, Fischer JS. Treatment of multiple sclerosis with methotrexate. In: Goodkin DE, Rudick RA (eds.). *Treatment of Multiple Sclerosis: Advances in Trial Design, Results, and Future Perspectives.* London: Springer, 1996, 251–287.

3. Weinstein A, Schwid SR, Schiffer RB, et al. Neuropsychologic status in multiple sclerosis after treatment with glatiramer. *Arch Neurol* 1999;56(3):319–324. Erratum in: *Arch Neurol* 2004;61(8):1284.

4. Pliskin NH, Hamer DP, Goldstein DS, et al. Improved delayed visual reproduction test performance in multiple sclerosis patients receiving interferon beta-1b. *Neurology* 1996;47(6):1463–1468.

5. Barak Y, Achiron A. Effect of interferon-beta-1b on cognitive functions in multiple sclerosis. *Eur Neurol* 2002;47(1):11–4.

6. Langdon D. Cognitive subgroup of the European Trial of Betaferon in SPMS. Effect of Betaferon on cognitive function: results of the European trial on secondary progressive multiple sclerosis. Poster presented at the annual meeting of ECTRIMS, Toulouse, France, September, 2000.

7. Fischer JS, Priore RL, Jacobs LD, et al. Neuropsychological effects of interferon beta-1a in relapsing multiple sclerosis. Multiple Sclerosis Collaborative Research Group. *Ann Neurol* 2000 Dec;48(6):885–92.

8. Bever CT Jr, Anderson PA, Leslie J, et al. Treatment with oral 3,4 diaminopyridine improves leg strength in multiple sclerosis patients: results of a randomized, double-blind, placebo-controlled, crossover trial. *Neurology* 1996;47(6):1457–1462.

9. Smits RC, Emmen HH, Bertelsmann FW, et al. The effects of 4–aminopyridine on cognitive function in patients with multiple sclerosis: a pilot study. *Neurology* 1994;44(9):1701–1705.

10. Rossini PM, Pasqualetti P, Pozzilli C, et al. Fatigue in progressive multiple sclerosis: results of a randomized, double-blind, placebo-controlled, crossover trial of oral 4-aminopyridine. *Mult Scler* 2001;7(6):354–358.

11. Cohen RA, Fisher M. Amantadine treatment of fatigue associated with multiple sclerosis. *Arch Neurol* 1989;46(6):676–680.

12. Sailer M, Heinze HJ, Schoenfeld MA, et al. Amantadine influences cognitive processing in patients with multiple sclerosis. *Pharmacopsychiatry* 2000;33(1):28–37.

13. Geisler MW, Sliwinski M, Coyle PK, et al. The effects of amantadine and pemoline on cognitive functioning in multiple sclerosis. *Arch Neurol* 1996;53(2):185–188.

14. Rammohan KW, Rosenberg JH, Lynn DJ, et al. Efficacy and safety of modafinil (Provigil) for the treatment of fatigue in multiple sclerosis: a two centre phase 2 study. *J Neurol Neurosurg Psychiatry* 2002; 72(2):179–183.

15. Wilken, JA, Wallin MT, Sullivan, SL, et al. An interim analysis of combination therapy (Modafinil [Provigil®] + Interferon ß-1a [AVONEX®]) in the treatment of cognitive problems in patients with relapsing-remitting MS. Poster presented at the annual meeting of the Consortium of Multiple Sclerosis Centers, Toronto, Canada, June, 2004.

16. Leo GJ, Rao SM. Effects of intravenous physostigmine and lecithin on memory loss in multiple sclerosis. *J Neuro Rehab* 1988;2:123–129.

17. Unverzagt FW, Rao SM, Antuono P. Oral physostigmine in the treatment of memory loss in multiple sclerosis. *J Clin Exp Neuropsychol* 1991;13:74 (Abstract).

18. Greene YM, Tariot PN, Wishart H, et al. A 12–week, open trial of donepezil hydrochloride in patients with multiple sclerosis and associated cognitive impairments. *J Clin Psychopharmacol* 2000;20(3): 350–356.

19. Krupp AB, Elkins LE, Scott SR, et al. Donepezil for the treatment of memory impairments in multiple sclerosis. Presentation at the American Academy of Neurology 51st Annual Meeting, Toronto, Canada, April, 1999: A137.

20. Krupp LB, Christodoulou C, Melville P, et al. Donepezil improved memory in multiple sclerosis in a randomized clinical trial. *Neurology* 2004;63(9):1579–1585.

21. Oliveri RL, Sibilia G, Valentino P, et al. Pulsed methylprednisolone induces a reversible impairment of memory in patients with relapsing-remitting multiple sclerosis. *Acta Neurol Scand* 1998;97(6):366–369.

22. Patzold T, Schwengelbeck M, Ossege LM, et al. Changes of the MS functional composite and EDSS during and after treatment of relapses with methylprednisolone in patients with multiple sclerosis. *Acta Neurol Scand* 2002;105(3):164–168.

23. Richards TL, Lappin MS, Acosta-Urquidi J, et al. Double-blind study of pulsing magnetic field effects on multiple sclerosis. *J Altern Complement Med* 1997;3(1):21–29. Erratum in: *J Altern Complement Med* 1997;3(2):205.

24. Geisler MW, Gaudino EA, Squires NK, et al. Cooling and multiple sclerosis: cognitive and sensory effects. *J Neuro Rehab* 1996;10:17–21.

25. Corey-Bloom J, Kenney C, Norman M. Ginkgo biloba slows cognitive decline in patients with multiple sclerosis. Presentation at the American Academy of Neurology 54th Annual Meeting, Denver, Colorado, April, 2002.

26. Gillson G, Richard TL, Smith RB, Wright JV. A double-blind pilot study of the effect of Prokarin on fatigue in multiple sclerosis. *Mult Scler* 2002;8(1):30–35.

27. Sullivan MJL, Dehoux E, Buchanan DC. An approach to cognitive rehabilitation in multiple sclerosis. *Can Jour Rehab* 1989;3(2):77–85.

28. Jønsson A, Korfitzen EM, Heltberg A, et al. Effects of neuropsychological treatment in patients with multiple sclerosis. *Acta Neurol Scand* 1993;88(6):394–400.

29. Rodgers D, Khoo K, MacEachen M, et al. Cognitive therapy for multiple sclerosis: a preliminary study. *Altern Ther Health Med* 1996;2(5): 70–74.

30. Shepko AG, Hollenbeck MA. Comparison of treatment duration for remediation of memory impairment in individuals with multiple sclerosis. *Mult Scler* 1997;3:208 (Abstract).

31. Ricker J. Memory retraining in multiple sclerosis. NMSS Pilot Project Research Report. 2002

32. Allen DN, Goldstein G, Heyman RA, Rondinelli T. Teaching memory strategies to persons with multiple sclerosis. *J Rehab Res Dev* 1998; 35(4):405–410.

33. Benedict RH, Shapiro A, Priore R, et al. Neuropsychological counseling improves social behavior in cognitively-impaired multiple sclerosis patients. *Mult Scler* 2000;6(6):391–396.
34. LaRocca NG, Caruso L, Kalb RC, et al. Comprehensive rehabilitation of cognitive dysfunction in multiple sclerosis. *Mult Scler* 1998; 4:460 (Abstract).
35. Foley FW, Dince WM, Bedell JR, et al. Psychoremediation of communication skills for cognitively impaired persons with multiple sclerosis. *J Neuro Rehab* 1994;8(4):165–176.
36. Plohmann AM, Kappos L, Ammann W, et al. Computer assisted retraining of attentional impairments in patients with multiple sclerosis. *J Neurol Neurosurg Psychiatry* 1998;64(4):455–462.
37. Mendozzi L, Pugnetti L. Computer assisted memory retraining of patients with multiple sclerosis. *Ital J Neurol Sci* 1998;19:S431–S438.
38. Solari A, Motta A, Mendozzi L, et al. CRIMS Trial. Computer-aided retraining of memory and attention in people with multiple sclerosis: a randomized, double-blind controlled trial. *J Neurol Sci* 2004; 15;222(1–2):99–104. Erratum in: *J Neurol Sci* 2004;15;224(1–2):113.
39. Chiaravalloti ND, Demaree H, Gaudino EA, DeLuca J. Can the repetition effect maximize learning in multiple sclerosis? *Clin Rehab* 2003;17(1):58–68.
40. Chiaravalloti ND, DeLuca J, Moore NB, Ricker JH. Treating learning impairments improves memory performance in multiple sclerosis: a randomized clinical trial. *Mult Scler* 2005;11(1):58–68.
41. Lincoln NB, Dent A, Harding J, et al. Evaluation of cognitive assessment and cognitive intervention for people with multiple sclerosis. *J Neurol Neurosurg Psychiatry* 2002;72(1):93–98.
42. Demaree HA, Gaudino EA, DeLuca J, Ricker JH. Learning impairment is associated with recall ability in multiple sclerosis. *J Clin Exp Neuropsychol* 2000;22(6):865–873.
43. Birnboim S, Miller A. Cognitive strategies application of multiple sclerosis patients. *Mult Scler* 2004;10(1):67–73.
44. Oken BS, Kishiyama S, Zajdel D, et al. Randomized controlled trial of yoga and exercise in multiple sclerosis. *Neurology* 2004 8;62(11): 2058–2064.

CHAPTER **6**

STRATEGIES FOR MANAGING COGNITIVE CHANGES

Nicholas LaRocca, PhD, and Lauren Caruso, PhD

•••

This chapter is designed to help you develop effective, individualized tools for dealing with multiple-sclerosis (MS)-related cognitive changes. Our basic assumptions are that one size does not fit all, and that common sense strategies applied in a consistent fashion can make a big difference. As you work your way through this chapter, you will find that we have not provided prepackaged tools. Instead, we provide instructions and easy-to-follow examples that will enable you to develop your own strategies to fit your style, abilities, and situation. Clinical experience has taught us that no one perfect system exists that works equally for all. Instead, you need to think about what works for you and then draw up a strategy that suits your own unique needs. So, this chapter will help you to gain an understanding of what you must consider to develop and implement cognitive strategies. Although developing your own strategies may seem more complicated and time-consuming than having them handed to you, being able to develop them yourself, in a way that fits your own style, will afford you a measure of independence in coping with cognitive changes.

When we talk about "strategies" or "tools," we are not referring to things that will reverse memory loss or speed up information processing. Instead, we are looking to "compensate" or "substitute" in some way for a function that is not working as well as it should. For example, if you find that you cannot keep all your social and work-related appointments in your head (and who can?), you might use an appointment book or personal digital assistant (PDA) to keep track of them. Using an appointment book or PDA is a compensatory strategy that utilizes substitution in that it substitutes a written or electronic record of appointments for those that might otherwise fade from memory. This type of strategy might not actually help you to "remember" an appointment, but it will make it more likely that you will appear at the right time and in the right place.

KEY ELEMENTS OF STRATEGY BUILDING AND MAINTENANCE

Now down to business. Several key elements are necessary to developing and using strategies to counter cognitive changes. We summarize them here, then refer back to them as we discuss a number of examples of strategies.

- **Determine what kinds of problems you are experiencing.** This can be accomplished through your own personal insight as well as objective testing. For example, if it's a memory problem, does it involve forgetting appointments, forgetting where you have left things, not remembering names, or some combination of these?
- **Try to sort out your strong and weak points.** For example, are you a well-organized person, but absent-minded?
- **Convince yourself that it's OK to do things differently than you did in the past.** Maybe you never needed to use a shopping list in the past, but now you can't remember even small numbers of items when you go to the store. Be willing to shift gears and use a more effective strategy—this will work far better than clinging to your old ways of doing things that are no longer effective.
- **Think about your personal "style"** of doing things; that is, how you operate in everyday life and which types of approaches tend to work best for you. For example, are you comfortable using high-tech gadgets or do you find that good old paper and pencil works best for you?
- **Design a strategy to address the problem.** It may take some trial and error and brainstorming to come up with a plan that satisfies you and solves the problem.
- **Keep it simple.** Developing a strategy that is more complicated than the problem is generally not helpful. Try to design your

strategy so that it is as simple as possible while still addressing the problem at hand. Break complex tasks into "bite-sized" pieces that are more manageable.

- **Tweak.** Like new software or a design for a new airplane, cognitive strategies may need to be revised based on actual experience. So, try out your strategy for a while, determine which parts are working well and which parts are not working well, and tweak. Revise your strategy based on experience and go on from there.

- **Adapt your strategy based on changing conditions.** A strategy that works well today might not work as well if your situation changes next month or next year. So, be on the lookout for changes in your life or your MS that may require revisions in your strategy.

- **Use the strategy consistently.** How many times have you heard someone say: "I had the appointment written down, but I forgot to look at my calendar." The strategies that you develop will only make a difference if they are applied consistently. There is no one "perfect" strategy, and the strategy that you can use consistently will probably be best for you.

- **Evaluate periodically.** On a regular basis, ask yourself, "How am I doing?" This periodic check-up can help to identify glitches that occur, such as a strategy that is no longer working as well as it used to. The check-up can also tell you if you are no longer using your strategy as consistently as you once were. In addition, you might also find that you have some new ideas to make a strategy that is working fairly well work even better. The bottom line in all of this, of course, is: Does the strategy actually make a difference in my everyday life?

- **Don't ignore your emotions.** How you feel and the stresses in your life can affect your ability to use your cognitive abilities. Dealing effectively with cognitive changes may therefore require attention to what's going on in your life on the emotional front.

- **Work with someone.** Although it is possible to do all the above on your own, it will be enhanced by working with someone—a professional, if possible—or even a peer, if professional help is not feasible. Whether it's an exercise program, a diet, or cognitive strategies, having the encouragement and support of another person can go a long way toward keeping you on track. Moreover, professional help can speed the process and open up opportunities that might be hard to realize on your own.

EXAMPLES

The following examples are presented to give you a better idea of how the process of strategy building and maintenance works. Some of the problems described may apply to you and others might not. Some of these strategies may be close to what you need to help you deal with cognitive problems, while others would need to be changed significantly. We strongly encourage you to go through all the steps outlined earlier to ensure that the strategies you use are tailored to your needs and situation. This is a process that you can undertake yourself to some extent. However, your results may be enhanced if you can work with a professional such as a neuropsychologist, speech pathologist, or occupational therapist.

Each example is labeled with the cognitive function that is the primary target of the strategy to be described. Of course, the workings of the mind are not quite that simple, and most things that we do in daily life involve a number of cognitive functions simultaneously. Once you get the hang of developing and implementing strategies, you will find that you may have several running at once, complementing one another like the members of a basketball team. However, to develop and refine strategies, it is helpful to identify individual functions that have been affected by MS and to come up with strategies to deal with each of these.

Shopping List (Memory)

As our first example, let's say that MS appears to have affected your memory in several ways. One way in which it has affected your memory is the increased difficulty that you have when you go grocery shopping. Even when you just need a few items, you find that you can't remember these and almost always wind up having to go back to the store for one or more forgotten items. You decide that you need a shopping list, even for short trips. Your best friend tells you about her approach. She keeps a sort of universal list of dozens of groceries on her computer and, when she needs something, she copies and pastes the item into a Word document. This works for your friend, because she is on her computer most of the day doing e-mail, surfing the Web, and the like. However, when you think about this, you just can't picture yourself doing it. The whole thing sounds unnecessarily complicated. On your next trip to the supermarket, you pick up a "handy checklist" provided by the store, which allows you to check items that you need. You find, however, that many items on the list you never buy, for example, canned vegetables, and that a lot of things you buy regularly are not there. Moreover, so many items are on the list that you are sure it will only serve to confuse you as you try to navigate among the aisles.

You finally decide that the best approach for you is just a simple, old-fashioned list that you keep near the fridge and that you take with you, even if you only need a few items. You find that this simple, classic approach works pretty well, and your trips for just a few things are less likely to come up short. However, as you use the list, you begin to notice that a problem arises that you did not anticipate. Although you are very consistent about taking the list to the store and looking at it when you are there, you find that you often forget to put things on the list in the first place. As a result, you may return from the store with everything on the list only to discover that you are out of an item that you forgot to write on the list before leaving the house.

So you decide that some revisions are needed, and you start to think about how to tackle this problem. Your friend's computerized list still does not appeal to you, nor does the supermarket's standard checklist. However, you decide that these two approaches do have one thing in common that you might be able to adapt to your needs. Rather than forcing you to think of what you need, these two approaches provide a "pool" of items and thus remind you of items that you might otherwise overlook. You decide to make up your own list of all the items that you buy on a regular basis and post it on the fridge next to the pad you use for making your shopping list. Now, before you go to the store, you take a quick glance at your "master list" and make sure there isn't anything that you have forgotten to add to your shopping list. You find that this simple addition to your strategy works well, and it is rare that you return from the supermarket to find that some needed item never made it home with you.

Packing List (Memory)

You travel for business on a pretty regular basis and make family trips four or five times a year. Recently, you have noticed that packing has become a hassle. When it comes time to pack, you find yourself chaotically grabbing things at random and in no particular order. The whole process takes longer and is more stressful than you ever remember it being. Moreover, you have begun to forget little things, such as ties on one trip, socks on another, and your medication on another. A friend in your MS support group suggests that you make

Things to be Packed	
✔	Shoes
✔	Socks
✔	Underwear
✔	Shirts
✔	Slacks
✔	Ties
✔	Medications
	Toiletries kit
	Travel documents and ID
	Etc.
Other Things to Do	
✔	Arrange car service
	Change phone message
	Etc

FIGURE 6.1. A simple packing list.

up a packing list (Figure 6.1) with all the items you usually need to take, and check things off on this list every time you pack for a trip.

You try this and find that the whole process of packing goes a lot more smoothly. However, you still find other trip-related details that are at risk of falling through the cracks, such as calling ahead for a car service to take you to the airport. Once you incorporate these items into your packing list, you find that travel has become a much more enjoyable process.

Family Calendar (Memory)

You have had MS for 20 years, and it has affected a number of aspects of your life. Walking is difficult, and you pretty much rely on a motorized scooter to move about outside your house. Your vision has been moderately affected as well, and you long ago stopped driving. Fatigue is a big issue, and you find that you run out of steam by mid-afternoon, even on days when you have not been too busy. In addition, MS has affected your memory and, unless you write things down, you are pretty likely to forget them. In spite of these changes, you continue to be the nerve center for your family, and your husband and two teenage daughters rely on you to keep things running smoothly.

You are happy with your role and feel that you do it well. However, in the last few months, some problems have arisen. Yours is an active family, and you have been having trouble coordinating family events. Friction has developed because family members talk to you about their activities and plans but you are having trouble remembering it all. A major row erupted last week when your daughters told you that they were going to a basketball game the same day that your parents were coming over for dinner. The girls insisted that they had told you 2 weeks ago about this special tournament, but you denied having heard anything about it. After the shouting ends, you decide that you need to do something about these schedules.

You talk about this experience in your weekly support group, and one of the other members reports going through the same sort of problems. Her solution was to set up a family calendar. You listen carefully and decide to adopt this solution. At the local office supply store, you buy a large month-by-month calendar, the kind used in offices. You sit down with the whole family and explain that, due to your memory problems and the busy lives of everyone in the family, just talking about activities doesn't work. You ask for their help by making sure that they enter on the calendar any activities or appointments that they have outside of the normal work or school day. There is some grumbling at first from your daughters, who complain about living in a "police state" and how they are just too busy to stop and write every time they make a move. However, with support from your husband they finally come to understand that this is something that will not only help you but also help to avoid unnecessary conflicts in scheduling. Things are a bit rough the first month and everyone forgets to put down some items. However, after 2 or 3 months, it all becomes second nature, and everyone is able to see the benefits. Your memory has not improved, but your trusty family calendar never forgets.

Project Flowchart (Sequencing)

During the last couple of years, you have found it frustrating to get projects completed, even small ones like organizing a photo album. Everything seems so complicated. It is hard for you to keep track of all the details, including the sequence in which things need to take place and the deadlines for getting things done. A typical experience might be that you are working on one aspect of a project and realize that some other aspect of it actually needed to be completed first. Another common experience is that you start on a task that is part of a larger project, and wind up delaying your co-workers because you didn't allow yourself enough time. When such things happen, you become really anxious and your performance deteriorates even further.

Someone at work tells you about a couple of software programs that offer project management. You look at these, but they seem so complicated that you feel they would only make the problem worse. So you are at a loss as to what to do. You share your concern with your sister, whom you consider a model of organization and efficiency. She tells you that early in her working career she often found herself floundering when trying to get projects done—backtracking, missing deadlines, and the like. As the two of you talk, she pulls out a couple of what she calls "project flowcharts." These provide a template for breaking projects up into discrete and manageable parts, laying out the sequence in which things need to get done, estimating how long it will take to complete each part, and establishing deadlines for each task. The whole thing looks so simple and straightforward that you wonder why you didn't think of it yourself.

Your sister helps you to set up a flowchart for a project that you were assigned at work—finding a new vendor for Internet service. The next day, armed with your flowchart, you start the process of identifying vendors. You have a great sense of relief because, for the first time in weeks, you don't feel as though things are spinning out of control. During the next few days, you continue to use the flowchart but notice a few glitches. When you and your sister drew up the chart, you broke the project down into a few discrete tasks. However, you find that many details are involved in each task, and you are overlooking them as you work your way through the project. Working with your sister again, you revise the flowchart, breaking the project down into smaller tasks and adding more detail. This turns out to work well, and the project is completed successfully on time and with much less in the way of hassles and anxiety.

Bill-Paying System (Sequencing)

Paying bills was never exactly your favorite thing to do. However, you always did it in a timely fashion and without too much muss and fuss. However, 15 years of living with MS seems to have taken its toll on your ability to keep things organized and get the bills out on time. Unpaid bills seem to get scattered all about the house and, for the first time in your life, overdue notices are arriving—not for a lack of funds to pay them, but just because you don't seem to have a workable system. One day, when your adult son is visiting, you share your dilemma with him. He offers to take over your finances and handle everything for you. You are truly mortified by the thought and angrily inform him that you are perfectly capable of managing your own affairs, while hoping he will not detect the note of doubt in your voice.

You decide then and there that you have to do something about this situation but are not sure what to do. The next day you receive in the mail the listing of courses offered by your local community college's adult education program. One is a six-session course in "Organizing Your Personal Finances." That's for me, you tell yourself. Feeling just a little self-conscious, you sign up for the class and send in your fee. The class consists of fifteen people, mostly retirees, a couple of middle-aged folks like yourself, and a couple of thirtyish people. The instructor is a woman in her late fifties who teaches accounting at the local community college. On the first night of the class, the instructor has people introduce themselves and briefly state why they enrolled. You are pleasantly surprised to hear that a couple of the older students are there for the exact same reason you are—to get a better handle on keeping abreast of bill paying and such.

During one of the first sessions, the instructor helps you and the other students set up what she calls a personal bill-paying system (Figure 6.2). Each student uses it somewhat differently, but the basic principles are the same. For example, one of the students uses a computer to keep track of checks written, while you prefer the old-fashioned paper checkbook register. The system provides a step-by-step sequence to be followed from the time a bill arrives in the mail until the paid bill is filed. You and your fellow students begin to implement the system right away, so that during the remainder of the course you can report back and get feedback on your progress. You find at first that you tend to forget to implement the system or leave out a step. However, with encouragement from the instructor and your fellow students, who run into some of the same problems, little by little you become very consistent in applying the system. By the end of the course, you are once again a prompt and efficient bill payer. You tell your son that things are now working fine in regard to bill paying and let him know that if he ever needs any help managing his finances, you are there for him.

Character Cards (Reading)

You've always been an avid reader. However, you have found during the last couple of years that you are not able to enjoy reading as much as in the past. It's hard to keep track of the characters in nov-

BILL-PAYING SYSTEM
Open bills the day they arrive in the mail
Circle due date and add to "to be paid" folder
On a weekly basis, empty "to be paid" folder
Assemble the following materials: Bills from "to be paid" folder   Checkbook   Pen   Stamps   Return address labels   Calculator   Stapler   Most recent bank statement
Separate payment stub from remainder of bill
Write check
Record check in check register
If multiple pages, staple pages of bill together and set aside
Insert payment stub and check in envelope
Seal envelope, apply stamp and return address label
Return to step #5 for each remaining bill
When all bills are paid, file statements in your paid bills file drawer
Mail paid bills same day or next day at the latest

FIGURE 6.2. A personal bill-paying system.

els, and you tend to forget key elements of the plot line. In addition, you tend to lose your place in the book easily, even with just momentary distractions. Working with a psychologist, you consider several options. One idea is to write the characters names inside the back of the book. However, you hate jumping back and forth, and you find that even that brief interruption can leave you lost and confused. Instead, the psychologist suggests using a "character card" (Figure 6.3). This is a large index card on which you jot down the names of the main characters in the book and who they are. As you read, you use this card to help you keep track of your position on the page, so that if there is a momentary distraction, you can easily pick up where you left off. Moreover, when you do need to look up a character you don't remember, the names are right in front of you. Finally, the

CHARACTER'S NAME	WHO IS THIS?
George Smith	Alcoholic father
Shelia Smith	Long-suffering mom
Babs Smith	Overachieving daughter
Dr. Baker	Murder victim
Maloney	Sheriff
Sandra Diggs	Mom's best friend
Lou Sante	Ex-con friend of Dad's
Horace	Mysterious friend of Lou's
Maria Lopez	Wisecracking housekeeper

FIGURE 6.3. A character card to keep track of characters in a novel.

character card is your bookmark. Using the character card, you not only find that reading is once again fun, but you are better able to remember the characters, even without looking at the card.

Read, Write, and Talk (Reading)

One of your great joys in life has always been reading. Although you read an occasional novel, your real love is nonfiction that feeds your insatiable curiosity about the world. Whether it is science, history, politics, true crime—it's all a wonderful journey of discovery. However, shortly after you were diagnosed with MS, you discovered to your horror that you seemed to have developed what you referred to as a "non-stick" mind, like the coating on those pots that keeps food from sticking to them. You could still read easily, but nothing seemed to stick and the parts of a book that you read one day seemed to have disappeared into thin air by the following day.

You shared your concern with a friend who happens to be a speech pathologist. She had worked with patients with mild traumatic brain injury who had encountered exactly your sort of problem many times. Based on her experience, she suggested the following strategy. Always read with a notebook close by. As you read, try to pay attention to the major points presented by the author. Every few pages, jot down a few quick notes concerning the major points and a handful of supporting details (Figure 6.4). When you return to the book the next day or whenever, first review your notes, at least the most recent ones, before continuing. From time to time, sit down with a member of your family or a good (and patient) friend, and talk about what you have been reading.

TITLE: The Tipping Point		
AUTHOR: Malcolm Gladwell		
MAIN POINTS	**SUPPORTING DETAILS**	**SECONDARY POINTS**
Three rules of epidemics: law of the few, stickiness factor, power of context	Most started by a small number of persons. Simple changes can make a big difference in impact. Humans are very sensitive to their environment	There are usually many explanations for dramatic trends—all are usually part of a larger pattern. Some people are pivotal in starting trends

FIGURE 6.4. Note taking during reading helps you assimilate and retain what you have read.

You are at first horrified by the idea of using this strategy. Taking notes while you read would be like being in school again and would make reading a chore. Reviewing notes before continuing to read would feel like preparing for a pop quiz. And talking to family and friends about what you have been reading? Now that sounds like an effective way to get people to avoid you. However, you find that you are out of options and decide to give it all a try.

At first, you find it all hard to get used to, and taking notes from time to time makes reading feel very choppy—to the point where you fear this approach will just make things worse. After a couple of days, you are ready to give up but decide to talk to your friend the speech pathologist. She encourages you to stick with it for at least a week, and volunteers to be your audience each day by phone so that you can report what you have been reading. You go along with this and find that, after a few days, the process begins to feel more natural. More important, you discover to your delight that, for the first time in recent memory, you are able to remember what you have read from one day to the next. You explain to family members and friends what you are trying to do, why you need to talk to them about your readings, and you ask for their patience with this. Their reaction is universally something along the lines of "Of course I'm willing to help if I can." So conversations over dinner and at other times come to take on a more "educational" tone in addition to the usual gossip about family and friends not present. As time goes on, the whole process comes to be taken for granted by you and those around you. With occasional encouragement from your friend the speech pathologist, you continue the process and once again find that you enjoy reading.

Time Management Sheet (Organization)

You used to be a very well-organized person who got a lot of things done while still having time left over to "smell the flowers." As your MS has gotten worse, however, time has seemed to become a relentless enemy. As the day starts, you have good intentions and make out a schedule of what you want to do and when you plan to do it. However, by the end of the day, you generally find that only a few of your scheduled tasks have actually been accomplished and most of these much later than planned. You have no idea where all the time is going.

Working with an occupational therapist (OT), you draw up a different kind of schedule. In addition to a column for scheduled activities, a second column is there for "what really happened." Every hour, you enter in the second column what really happened during that time slot. After doing this for a few days, you begin to realize where all the time is going. First, you find that you scheduled too many activities and that activities scheduled for half an hour, for example, actually took an hour and a half. You also find that times occurred when you were scheduled to do one thing but ended up doing other things that weren't even on the list for that day. Some of these were unavoidable, like unexpected crises. However, it becomes clear to you that you tend to drift off into irrelevant activities and therefore don't accomplish what you set out to do. For example, on many days, you made long phone calls to friends when you were scheduled to do some other task.

With guidance from your OT, you first pare down the number of things that you attempt to accomplish in a given day. In addition, you make a list of the most frequent intrusions that have appeared in the "what really happened" column. You consult this list frequently to remind yourself to stay on track. You also refer to your time management sheet (Figure 6.5) frequently to make sure that you are not drifting.

At first it is a struggle and you tend to find yourself falling into the old habits. However, with encouragement and advice from your OT, you gradually reduce the intrusions to a minimal number. You find that you are accomplishing more than you have in years and feel much better about yourself.

94

TIME	SCHEDULED ACTIVITIES	WHAT REALLY HAPPENED
AM		
7:00	Get up and have breakfast	Pushed the snooze button
8:00	Tidy up	Ate breakfast
9:00	Call the bank	Called the bank (didn't tidy up!)
10:00	Run errands	Couldn't find list; got phone call
11:00	Run errands	Started late; ran into Debby
PM		
12:00	Pay bills	Grabbed a bite with Debby
1:00	Pay bills	Watched CNN
2:00	Rest	Paid some bills (missed my rest!)
3:00	Kids home	Homework and snack
4:00	Start dinner preparations	Call from Steven's teacher
etc.		Exhausted; 20 minute rest

FIGURE 6.5. Time management sheet.

Filing System (Organization)

You were never the world's most organized person, but in the past you were pretty much able to find things when you needed them, even if they were in sort of odd but "safe" places. However, MS seems to have taken its toll on that wonderful but quirky sense of organization that you used to keep in your head. Now you find that if you need a piece of paper—say your auto registration or your copy of last year's tax return—a major, frustrating hunt is in the offing. Moreover, your house has begun to look like the local recycling center with papers, bills (paid and unpaid), folders, and envelopes covering every surface.

While visiting your physical therapist for your weekly session, you bemoan the chaos that seems to have descended on your life. She suggests that you talk to her colleague, an occupational therapist in the same clinic, who is known to have a flare for organization. You set up an appointment to discuss the problem. The OT follows up with a home visit to better assess the damage, and together you develop a plan for a filing system to deal with paper and paperwork. You don't have much patience for complicated systems, so the two of you decide to keep it simple. You also have found that using color helps you to recognize things quickly and keep things straight, so the two of you decide to utilize color coding as much as possible in your system.

You have an old four-drawer filing cabinet in the basement, which you empty of such valuable items as your high school algebra homework and old copies of *People* magazine. The top drawer is devoted to current accounts such as gas, electric, telephone, and credit cards. It contains the paid bills from these various accounts as well as important documents from each, such as the contract for your cell phone. At the end of each year, you go through this drawer and dispose of anything that is no longer needed. The hanging folders in this drawer are blue. The next drawer contains information concerning your pension plan, bank accounts, and investments, including statements, cancelled checks, annual reports, and the like. This drawer is also purged at the end of each year. The hanging folders in this drawer are green. The third drawer is reserved for tax records, including federal and state tax returns, W-2s and 1099's when they arrive, real estate taxes, records of charitable donations, and the like. These records are retained for several years until your accountant tells you that they can be discarded. The hanging folders in this drawer are red. The bottom drawer is used for miscellaneous papers such as warranties, operating instructions for appliances, and what-have-you. The hanging folders in this drawer are yellow.

At the top of the filing cabinet, you place two trays. One tray is reserved for papers requiring action, such as bills that must be paid. The other is reserved for papers to be filed. In your kitchen, you establish a "paper port" consisting of a small bin where you drop any paperwork or mail that needs to be processed. Every day, you empty the paper port, go through the lot, and classify everything. To avoid having to examine papers more than once, you label each item with a colored dot to indicate which drawer or drawers it will eventually go into. While applying these dots involves an extra step, you find that it saves an enormous amount of time when you do your bill paying and filing. Each day, you transfer whatever is to be processed and/or kept to one of the two trays at the top of the filing cabinet and, once a week, you pay bills and do filing.

To-Do List (Prioritizing)

Over the years, as your MS has gotten worse, you have noticed that life seems to have gotten more complicated and harder to manage. You feel overwhelmed all the time by how much you have to do; you don't know where to begin, and things often don't get done on time or at all. Your doctor refers you to a neuropsychologist who does some cognitive testing and then works with you to address the issues

CALLS	PRIORITY	COMPLETED
Appointment with dentist	A	✔
Mom's doctor	A	✔
Cousin Bill re vacation house	B	✔
Furniture store re new sofa	C	
ERRANDS	**PRIORITY**	**COMPLETED**
Mail tax return	A	✔
Pick up prescription	A	✔
Pick up dry cleaning	B	✔
Return book to library	C	✔
Buy tickets for Sunday's game	C	
TASKS	**PRIORITY**	**COMPLETED**
Discuss Morgan account with Bev	A	✔
Meet with attorney	A	✔
Pay bills	B	
Replace furnace filter	B	
Throw out old magazines	C	

FIGURE 6.6. A prioritizing "to-do" list system.

with which you are having trouble in daily life. First and foremost for you is that "overwhelmed by too many things to do" feeling.

The two of you look at various options. Although you have a computer and use it daily, you really want something that you can carry around with you and write in on the fly. For this reason you pick a medium-sized, loose-leaf organizer that you find at your local office supply store. You and your psychologist set up four "zones" in the book to organize your "to-do's." These include Calls, Errands, Tasks, and Projects. The first three are things that can be done in less than a day, while projects tend to be longer-term; that is, generally taking more than a day to complete. On any given day, elements of one or more of the projects will be listed under calls, errands, or tasks. You set up a simple system of priorities: A—must be done by day's end; B—would like to do by day's end; and C—do today if all A and B to-do's have been completed (Figure 6.6).

Each morning, you review the to-do's from the previous day and set up your to-do's for today. You start with a clean page for the first three types of to-do's, while the projects page is retained. Periodically, you revise the projects page, crossing off completed projects and adding new ones. When things get really messy, you transfer the projects list to a fresh page.

As you set up the to-do's for the day, you assign an A, B, or C priority to each. As to-do's are completed during the day, you mark them as done. During the day, situations may arise in which you will have to add calls, errands, tasks, or projects to your lists. You do so as needed, and assign each an A, B, or C priority, being careful to balance these new items with the old so that you do not attempt to complete more in one day than is humanly possible.

Crisis Management (Prioritizing)

You have been working with your "to-do" list and prioritizing for a few weeks. You are happy with the way in which it has helped you to get the most important things done first while not totally neglecting the less pressing matters. However, one glitch exists in all of this that is familiar to anyone who has tried to prioritize activities. The problem is that the world does not stand still. You can start your day with a nice, neat set of to-do's that have been carefully prioritized. By mid-morning, however, at least one crisis has arisen at work that demands immediate attention. Moreover, it might not be the last. Although it is easy enough to say that crises go to the top of the to-do list, the whole process of integrating these emergent priorities tends to throw you off. You then find it hard to recover and continue working through the original priority list. When a crisis arises, should you drop whatever you are doing immediately and tend to the crisis? Should you try to finish a chunk of the to-do you are working on before side-stepping to deal with a crisis? Should you finish whatever you are working on before dealing with a crisis?

You discuss this dilemma with the neuropsychologist who helped you set up your to-do system. The two of you agree that every crisis is different and that Rule One for dealing with them is that you need to evaluate each one separately and decide on the appropriate course of action. In some cases, the only sensible thing to do will be to drop whatever you are doing and tend to the crisis. In other cases, you may have more or less breathing space to partially or completely finish whatever you had been working on. The two of you also discuss how best to set things up so that you can most efficiently pick up where you left off once the crisis has either passed or settled down somewhat. Here is the basic plan that you develop (Figure 6.7).

It doesn't take long before a crisis develops at work to test out this new system. The crisis in question turns out to be one needing

Quickly examine the "crisis" to determine if immediate action is needed or if any delay is feasible
Determine if someone else can either handle this crisis or assist you with it
Plan on when you will begin to address the crisis, e.g., immediately, an hour from now, tomorrow
Recruit assistance as needed
Before beginning work on the crisis, make a brief note clearly indicating where you were in any ongoing tasks and when you expect to be able to return to these
Carefully store any materials you had been working on with markers to indicate where you were working when you had to pause
If possible, refer the interrupted task to someone else for completion
Begin working on the crisis
When the crisis is resolved or settles down sufficiently, return to your to-do list, evaluate where you stand, and revise as needed
Resume work on interrupted tasks based on a revised to-do list with appropriate priorities

FIGURE 6.7. A crisis-management evaluation sheet.

immediate attention. You take about 10 minutes to go through the first few steps in your crisis management plan, including leaving your interrupted work in a state that will make it easy for you to pick up where you left off. Dealing with the crisis takes until about noon of the next day. At that point, you take a few minutes to update your to-do list for the day, making it a much truncated set of things to get done. You pick up where you left off the day before, and find that your preparations have made it relatively easy to quickly shift gears back to where you were. In the coming months, you find that you need to use the crisis management plan at least two or three times per week, usually for interruptions that last only an hour or two. In almost every case, the plan allows you to deal with the crisis, efficiently get back on track, and continue to work through those important but non-crisis to-do's.

Driving Directions (Visual–Spatial Abilities)

You have had MS for 12 years, and it does not seem to have had much effect on your ability to drive. Your reaction time and your ability to manage the accelerator, brakes, and steering are relatively unaffected. Night driving is not as easy as it used to be, but you avoid driving at night, leaving that to your husband. Your vision has been tested as OK for driving in general. However, finding your way around has become a major issue. You used to be able to find your way to places if you had been there once or twice. You now find that you can't quite picture the route in your head and, more often than not, you get confused and turn this way when you should have turned that way. Aside from the frustration of getting lost all the time and often showing up late, you find yourself in the embarrassing position of having to ask people for directions again and again. Your friends have begun to affectionately refer to you as the "lost soul."

During the last few weeks, you have been seeing a psychologist for help with depressive symptoms related to your MS and the recent death of your father. In the course of one of these sessions, you bemoan your driving snafus. Your psychologist suggests that the two of you work out a practical strategy to deal with the problem. You don't want to give up driving, and you can easily follow written directions, if you have them. The two of you work out a simple strategy. You use your computer to create a set of files containing driving directions for all the places that you visit on a regular basis. Whenever you have to go someplace new, you add these new directions to the files on your computer. You print out the set of directions in very large type that you will be able to see easily while you are driving. These are placed in a zippered plastic folder that stays put in your car, always at the ready. You make each set of directions as clear and as detailed as needed, with mileage, number of traffic lights, landmarks, and more. However, you avoid unnecessary and distracting detail. When you set out to go anywhere except the most familiar of places, you take out the appropriate sheet of directions, even if you think you are not going to need it. In this way you are prepared at a moment's notice to check, "Is that a right or a left?"

At first you are self-conscious about what you think of as your "dummy driver" file. However, one day, you and a friend are heading out together to visit a store a few miles away and she sees the file and all the neatly printed directions. She is so taken with it that she decides to make a similar file for herself and, before long, several in your circle of friends have their own versions. Moreover, while definitive proof is lacking, there is suspicion that even some of the husbands from time to time secretly peek at some of the driving directions, just to verify that they already know exactly where they are going.

Closet Organization (Visual-Spatial Abilities)

You love your walk-in closet. It was custom designed for you by one of those closet companies, and it makes the best use of space using several drawers, cabinets, and shelves in addition to the usual racks for hangers. It all worked well for you until recently. It is clear to you that MS has affected your ability to get and stay organized and to remember where things are. Your dream closet has turned into a minor nightmare in which, every time you enter, you descend into confusion and frustration, unable to find the item that you need and that you thought you had stored in such and such a place. The spaciousness of the closet now works to your detriment, because there are so many places where things can get lost, and the complexity of the different sections presents too many choices.

You had completed cognitive testing with a neuropsychologist due to this and other problems. including memory deficits and word-finding problems. You are now working with the neuropsychologist in a program of cognitive rehabilitation. The two of you set as one of your goals the development of a strategy to deal with the "closet from hell" problem. Your strategy encompasses the following features:

- Every item, whether clothes, shoes, accessories, or otherwise has a specific place assigned to it in the closet.
- Each item is returned to its assigned spot when not in use.
- Each section is clearly labeled for quick reference; for example, pants, jackets, scarves, shoes, belts, etc.
- A "map" of the closet is posted on the door that shows schematically each wall of the closet, with each section clearly indicated and labeled.
- Once a week, the closet is checked and any items out of place are moved to the correct section of the closet.

The whole idea of all this mapping and labeling at first struck you as annoyingly compulsive. You have found, however, that with just a bit of effort on your part, it is easy to maintain and has pretty much resolved the confusion and incessant hunting for things. Although you do backslide at times, and just throw things wherever, the weekly "tune-up" brings everything up to snuff again. Little by little, you get used to putting things where they belong because the rewards for doing so are so great. You and your closet are once again friends. Now, if it was just a little bit bigger....

Getting the Main Idea (Conceptual Reasoning)

You had always considered yourself to be pretty sharp, with a good mind to figure things out such as "whodunit" in mystery novels. After having MS for a few years, however, you have noticed that you often don't get the point in situations that would have been a breeze for you in the past. For example, you were watching a show on public TV that talked about changes in the world economy and their effects on the average person. When the show was over, you were at a loss to say what exactly the point was and, looking back, it all just seemed like a big jumble.

Because you have also experienced some other problems, such as occasional memory lapses, your doctor sent you for neuropsychological testing. When the testing was completed, scored, and interpreted, the neuropsychologist sat down with you to explain the results. She told you that the trouble you were having "figuring things out" is difficulty with "conceptual reasoning." The two of you then developed a program of cognitive rehabilitation to address the conceptual reasoning problem along with other deficits identified on the testing.

One way that you address the conceptual reasoning problem is through a technique called "getting the main idea." The neuropsychologist gives you a series of readings, mostly nonfiction. These are generally short, just a few pages at first. As you are reading each article, your job is to be on the lookout for the main idea and for details that support the main idea. The primary focus, however, is on getting the main idea. After you finish reading the article, you have to explain to the neuropsychologist what the main idea was and list at least four or five supporting details. The neuropsychologist then asks you a few questions about the article. After doing a few of these, the neuropsychologist asks you to begin to look for some of the secondary ideas as well. As time goes on, the articles become longer and more complex but, with practice, you find that you are getting better at it and your confidence is increasing. You find that you are applying your new-found skills not only to reading, but to other situations as well, such as conversations. Using this strategy on a consistent basis eventually makes a big difference in your ability to "figure things out." You still don't really understand the world economy, but the more you hear about it, the more you are convinced that you are not alone in this.

Puzzles and Proverbs (Conceptual Reasoning)

Although you have had MS for only a few years, you are surprised to find that it seems to have affected your mind. You tend to forget things much more than in the past, you often have trouble coming up with a word that you want to say, and, most puzzling, you find that you are having trouble understanding simple things like jokes, slogans, sayings, and the like. You tend to take things "literally" and often "don't get it" when people are using a figure of speech. For example, the other day, a friend said that, as a result of recent events in the stock market, he had "taken a bath." For a moment, you were confused by the seeming lack of connection between stocks and bathing but then remembered that "taking a bath" means a financial loss. You have also observed that you now have trouble sorting things into logical categories. For example, you had your house painted and, when you went to replace the books on your book-shelves, you had a lot of trouble coming up with a system for organizing them. You kept staring at the titles but just could not see a simple set of categories that you could use to separate them into groups.

After discussion with your psychotherapist, you go to see a neuropsychologist who completes testing and confirms what you had suspected concerning changes in several cognitive functions. She explains that your tendency at times to "not get it" and to have trouble sorting and categorizing is known as a deficit in conceptual reasoning. The two of you develop a plan for cognitive rehabilitation that includes a number of mental exercises that you do in the neuropsychologist's office, as well as several things that you can do on your own at home.

One of the homework assignments involves working with materials that challenge and hopefully sharpen your conceptual reasoning skills. These include proverbs, word puzzles, and some sections from an SAT practice workbook that cover skills such as analogies and conceptual reasoning. You work through all these on your own, and then in your rehab sessions, you review them with the neuropsychologist, explaining your understanding of each proverb, puzzle, or problem. As you do more and more of these, you find that your skills become sharper and the exercises become easier. As you gain confidence, you gradually take on more difficult material. At first, there does not seem to be much carryover to everyday life. However, as time goes on and your skills increase, you begin to find that your mind seems to work more quickly in day-to-day tasks, and you are better able to get the gist of things right away. The neuropsychologist explains that, although you have made progress, which is verified on testing, you will need to continue the exercises to maintain your newfound level of skill. You are happy to do so and have come to look forward to conquering the next puzzle or riddle.

DECISION-MAKING PROCESS
Define as clearly and simply as possible exactly what the decision is.
Gather relevant information and materials.
Organize the relevant information and materials and have them close at hand.
For each choice, list the pros and cons.
Eliminate any obviously undesirable choices.
Make a preliminary selection from the remaining choices.
Review your preliminary choice in terms of its pros and cons and any other considerations such as cost, feasibility, timeframe, etc.
Implement your choice.
Once the choice has been in effect for a period of time, review success of this choice compared to others.

FIGURE 6.8. A decision-making template.

Decision Template (Conceptual Reasoning)

You have relatively mild MS, at least to outward appearances—no cane, no wheelchair. However, it is the less visible effects that slow you down—trouble walking any considerable distance, devastating fatigue, and, strangest of all, indecision. Before you had MS, you were able to size up a situation quickly and come up with what was usually a pretty sound decision. However, in the last few months, you have found that even relatively minor decisions overwhelm you with details that you can't seem to sort out. A neuropsychological assessment confirms that you are experiencing difficulty with conceptual reasoning, speed of information processing, and memory. You start working with a neuropsychologist on a twice-weekly program of cognitive rehabilitation and stress management training.

Part of your cognitive rehabilitation involves what the neuropsychologist calls a "decision template" (Figure 6.8). This consists of a form and a set of procedures for using the form that take you step-by-step through the process of evaluating choices and arriving at a decision.

The first actual decision for which you implement the decision template is where to take the family on vacation. Preliminary discussion with your wife and kids narrows it down to two choices: Cape Cod or Florida. You make notes of what your wife and children say concerning each locale and, in addition, you gather tourist information about each area. You sit down with your notes and materials and list the pros and cons of each (Figure 6.9).

Cape Cod		Florida	
PRO	**CON**	**PRO**	**CON**
Close enough to drive there	Rental and food expensive	Good deals on flights and hotels	Crowded with lots of tourists
Quiet and relaxing	Limited activities for kids	Lots of activities for kids and grown-ups	Need a car to go anywhere
Beautiful surroundings	Don't know anyone there	Relatives live close by	*Relatives live close by
*You have never been there			This will be your third trip there
Nice climate in August			Very hot in August
Nice beaches			
*These points were identified as particularly important			

FIGURE 6.9. Using the decision-making template.

After completing the grid in which you list the pros and cons, you sit down with the rest of the family and review what you have come up with. Although some sentiment is in favor of Florida, eventually you arrive at a consensus that Cape Cod should be the choice. The grid helped you to identify two factors that more or less stood out from the rest. First, because you only have one week, you don't really want to spend it in an area where relatives reside. Although you are fond of your relatives, most of them at least, trying to visit all of them will cut into the time that you all want to just relax and get away from work, school, and home obligations. The second outstanding issue is the fact that none of you have ever visited Cape Cod. Seeing someplace new appeals to everyone in the family, and this tends to be the clincher.

The vacation is arranged, and you all pack off in the car to Cape Cod. Your analysis of pros and cons turns out to be pretty much on target—the Cape is expensive but beautiful. You are surprised, however, by the fact that your kids are not bored at all. They find other youngsters who are also vacationing with their parents and, all in all, you are quite happy with the way your decision has turned out. As time goes on, you use the decision template for a number of decisions having to do with household matters, personal finance, and work. It works quite well for you, and you wonder how you ever got along without it.

FINDING THE STRATEGIES
THAT WORK FOR YOU

We hope that this chapter has provided you with some good ideas. Given our basic assumption that one size doesn't fit all, your next step will be to go back to the beginning of this chapter and review the elements involved in developing strategies for yourself. Keep in mind that this will be a step-wise process requiring a trial-and-error approach, some patience, and a good deal of tweaking. The goal is to create strategies that work for you—given your particular challenges and environments (home, work, neighborhood) in which you want to be at your best.

CHAPTER 7

COGNITIVE VIGNETTES

Rosalind Kalb, PhD, and Lauren Caruso, PhD

• •

Having described multiple sclerosis (MS)-related cognitive changes in some detail—the functions that can be affected and the various ways to identify, measure, and treat them—and discussed the impact they can have on daily life, we now want to bring them to life. The following vignettes are designed to give you snapshots of the ways in which cognitive changes might impact an individual's everyday functioning, feelings of self-confidence and self-esteem, and relationships with others, as well as some suggested strategies for managing those changes. These vignettes are composite pictures of real people, but the details have been changed to protect their privacy. Each vignette includes a brief background description, a summary of the cognitive changes identified on neuropsychological testing, and a list of compensatory strategies for managing particular cognitive changes at home and at work.

Keep in mind as you read these that many people with MS experience no changes in their cognitive functioning. For those who do experience some change, most will have one or two areas of relatively mild deficit; in rare instances, a person may have so many deficits of such severity that his or her daily functioning is severely impacted. The people in these vignettes are each dealing with common types and combinations of problems. What becomes clear in these real-life situations is that cognitive challenges affect different people in different ways, depending on how the changes they are experiencing interact with their roles and responsibilities at home and at work.

The recommended strategies are representative of those that might be used to address the problems described, but are not meant to be an exhaustive list or a substitute for professional advice. In many instances, the strategies can be used without professional help; working with a cognitive rehabilitation specialist, however, will help to ensure that you are using the strategies best suited to the problems you are having, and that you are using them in the most effective way. In other words, the specialist functions like a coach—making recommendations that are specific to your particular situation, monitoring their impact, and revising the strategies as needed.

LAURA—CHEF

Background

Laura, a 47-year-old chef, is employed in an upscale restaurant. She was diagnosed with MS nine years ago, but believes—based on mild visual and sensory symptoms that would appear sporadically over the years—that she has actually had the disease for longer than that. She has been on a disease-modifying agent since shortly after her diagnosis was confirmed, and her physical symptoms have remained fairly stable for the past few years. Laura's current symptoms include fatigue, spasms in her legs, episodes of blurred vision, and urinary frequency and urgency.

For the past few months, Laura has been finding it increasingly difficult to coordinate the activities of her staff, track what is happening in the bustling kitchen, and focus on her individual tasks. These changes have begun to eat away at her self-esteem, and she finds herself feeling more self-conscious and less confident in her interactions with others. She is aware that she feels and functions less well when she is tired and is increasingly bothered by the heat of the kitchen. As the restaurant has become more successful, and the pace of activity has accelerated, Laura has found it harder to keep up. Although very creative, Laura is having more trouble visualizing the physical presentation of the new entrees she tries to design. As a result, those aspects of her work that she used to find most enjoyable have now become major sources of stress.

Test Results

Laura's estimated *premorbid* (prior to MS) IQ was in the high average to superior range; she graduated in the top third of her class in culinary school. Her language skills and memory have been unaffected by MS. While she always had good organizational skills, it was her passion for cooking that ensured her success. Her current deficits, including impairments in information-processing speed, ability to shift between tasks, sequencing, and visual spatial organization, account for the types of problems she has begun to have in her everyday life. In fact, Laura felt quite validated by these results, since they explained and confirmed what she had been experiencing on a day-to-day basis.

Compensatory Strategies

Laura has developed some organizational strategies to relieve the pressure and stress in the busy kitchen. She has a daily schedule posted on the wall that she and her staff can all see, and has created templates and lists for aspects of her job that are the same from one day to the next. These tools allow her to perform complex daily tasks without having to plan and organize the necessary steps each time. Laura has also made it her goal to focus on a limited array of tasks that utilize her strengths. She has begun to delegate some of the organizational aspects of her job—which leaves her free to focus more on the creative aspects she enjoys—and works with another chef on the design of the physical presentation of new entrees. For those entrees that are her particular specialty, she has created design templates that she and her staff can follow. Although Laura was initially quite sad about having to make these changes, she feels less stressed over the course of the day, and finds that she enjoys the increased collaboration with others.

To deal with the intense heat in the kitchen, Laura has begun wearing a cooling vest, and she makes sure that she always has a glass of ice water at hand. She also schedules in a brief rest between the lunch and dinner hours.

As the restaurant gets busier and more fast-paced, Laura may find it increasingly difficult to cope with her slowed processing speed. At that time, she may need to consider transitioning to a smaller or less busy restaurant, working part-time (choosing either the lunch or dinner hour), or moving out of the restaurant setting into a teaching role.

KAREN—HIGH SCHOOL TEACHER

Background

Karen is a 42-year-old high school social studies teacher. She was diagnosed with MS 10 years ago. Her symptoms include mild sensory changes in her face and limbs that come and go, occasional bouts of fatigue, particularly in hot weather, and cognitive changes. While typically mild and manageable, her cognitive symptoms get significantly worse when she has an exacerbation. In fact, Karen's exacerbations are primarily cognitive, with the symptoms lasting two to three months.

Normally a highly enthusiastic, articulate, and expressive teacher, Karen finds during exacerbations that she is often at a loss for words as well as thoughts. She is easily distracted by activity in the classroom or the hallway, which causes her to lose her train of thought during lectures or class discussions. If a student interrupts a lecture to ask a question, Karen has difficulty picking up where she left off. She frequently finds that words are "on the tip of her tongue" but out of reach. Because of problems with divided attention, Karen can't write on the blackboard and lecture at the same time.

Karen has noticed that exacerbations also affect her moods. She experiences feelings of depression and anxiety about the exacerbation that seem to make the cognitive symptoms worse—or at least feel worse. Karen is used to functioning at a very high level; even subtle changes in her cognition, that others wouldn't notice, threaten her self-confidence and increase her anxiety. Because each exacerbation can last many weeks, Karen is relieved that their frequency and severity have lessened since she changed disease-modifying therapies about six years ago.

Test Results

Karen's premorbid IQ is estimated to have been in the superior range. Her strengths lie in her high intelligence, strong knowledge base in her subject area, and good organizational skills. During exacerbations, she experiences slowed information processing, verbal memory deficits, and problems with complex attention tasks and executive functions. Karen's functioning in every area returns to near normal during periods of remission.

Compensatory Strategies

Following the first exacerbation that caused Karen significant cognitive problems, she decided to explain to her students about MS and the problems with thinking, attention, and word-finding that sometimes occurred. Karen's reasons for sharing this information with the students were two-fold. She hoped that by telling them what was going on, it would relieve some of the pressure on her, thereby reducing the anxiety that seemed to make the cognitive problems worse. In addition, she hoped to enlist the students' assistance. During a subsequent episode that year, Karen engaged the help of her students for word finding—much to her amusement, the kids saw it as a new form of charades—and writing on the blackboard. They also helped her get back on track if she temporarily lost her train of thought. These strategies were so effective that Karen decided to talk about her MS at the beginning of each new school year, so that her students would be "prepped" in the event that she needed their assistance during the year.

During exacerbations, Karen also prepares "cue cards" for her lectures, and takes a few minutes ahead of each class to "rehearse" in her head the general gist of the lecture she is going to give. She sits during class to conserve energy for thinking and lecturing—a significant challenge for a teacher who is used to being on her feet and moving around among her students. The school has put an air conditioner in her classroom to help combat fatigue caused by the heat.

The combination of all these strategies has relieved much of Karen's anxiety, which in turn has made the cognitive symptoms feel less severe. Counseling has helped her deal with the emotional turmoil surrounding her MS, and also provides brain-storming sessions for new and creative compensatory strategies.

KEVIN—COLLEGE STUDENT

During his senior year of high school, Kevin—now a 20-year-old college student—thought he was suddenly "getting stupid." He was diagnosed with MS one year later, following a bout of optic neuritis and double vision. Kevin is now in his sophomore year and planning to major in European languages.

Except for late afternoon fatigue, Kevin's early physical symptoms are in remission. His cognitive symptoms, however, continue to be a problem. Kevin is having trouble keeping up with the lectures and class discussion, especially toward the end of a difficult class and at the end of the day. As a result, he is very reluctant to express an opinion or ask questions. He has difficulty screening out distractions, such as classmates talking or shuffling papers. He finds that he is not able to learn and remember new material as well as he did in the past, and his philosophy course is posing particular challenges because of the abstract concepts involved. During exams, Kevin finds that he is generally able to think through and respond to the questions, but needs more time than the other students. All of Kevin's problems are worse when he is having an exacerbation.

Kevin's parents are worried and think he should be at home where they can look after him. His neurologist, however, is encouraging him and them to utilize the support services available at school so that he can complete his education, enjoy the complete college experience, and learn to manage his MS independently. Even though Kevin's symptoms are primarily cognitive at this time, the neurologist has started him on a disease-modifying therapy in an effort to reduce the frequency and severity of his exacerbations and slow the progression of his cognitive symptoms. Kevin has experienced some significant bouts of depression and pessimism about his future; he worries about how the disease might progress, and wonders if he will be able to have a "normal" life.

Test Results

Kevin's premorbid IQ is estimated in the high average range. He was an A/B student in high school, graduating in the top quarter of his class, and showed a particular talent for mastering languages. Kevin's English language skills and visual memory remain strong. However, learning new vocabulary and mastering foreign grammar rules are now very difficult for him. His current deficits include impairments in verbal memory, information-processing speed, conceptual reasoning, divided attention, and some mild problems with planning and prioritizing.

Compensatory Strategies

Kevin decided to reduce his course load to give himself a chance to develop some effective compensatory strategies. In consultation with a cognitive rehabilitation specialist, he developed a study planner to help him schedule his study hours more effectively. He takes advantage of the times in the day when he is most rested and alert, takes frequent breaks, and doesn't try to focus for too long on any one subject. These strategies combine to reduce his cognitive fatigue. Kevin also tries to maintain good sleep hygiene (getting to bed at a consistent time and sleeping for a sufficient number of hours)—never an easy goal for a college student.

At the suggestion of his neurologist and the cognitive remediation specialist, Kevin asked for some accommodations from the office of disability at the school. He tapes all his lectures so that he can re-listen to any of them as needed. This helps him "overlearn" the material until he feels that the facts and concepts are at his fingertips. Kevin has also been given permission to take untimed exams in a room by himself.

Kevin is definitely a child of the computer age. He has discovered that his electronic organizer and computer provide many opportunities to substitute organization for memory. With some assistance from the cognitive rehabilitation specialist, he has created a filing system on his computer that helps him stay organized, and he keeps lists of everything he has to do—with an alarm system in his organizer that beeps him with reminders.

The remediation specialist also provided Kevin with some computer-based exercises that may improve his attention and concentration, and encouraged Kevin to use computer games and puzzles to improve his visual-spatial skills, sequencing abilities, and processing speed. In addition, the specialist encouraged Kevin to capitalize on his visual memory skills by drawing pictures or diagrams of the vocabulary and grammar rules he is trying to remember.

At the suggestion of his neurologist, Kevin is seeing a counselor at the school. He was found to have a mild depression, which is thus far manageable with regular therapy sessions focusing on problem-solving and management of daily activities. He and the counselor have agreed that if the depressive symptoms increase, he will be referred for a psychiatric evaluation to determine if an antidepressant medication is needed.

FRAN—MOTHER AND ATTORNEY

Background

Fran is a 45-year old attorney with two children, aged 16 and 18 years. She was diagnosed with MS 15 years ago, and started on a disease-modifying therapy when they first became available. She uses an electric scooter and an accessible van. She has weakness and spasticity in her legs, occasional painful sensory symptoms in her trunk and arms, and fatigue. After years of dealing only with physical symptoms, Fran is aware that her thinking and ability to process information are not as agile as they used to be. She is having trouble keeping track of everything she needs to remember at home and at work. If, while working on one thing, she is called upon to focus on something else, she finds it hard to shift gears or remember what she was doing when she was interrupted. Fran also experiences significant cognitive fatigue when she tries to focus on a particular mental task for a long period of time. She is aware that her cognition is worse during her occasional exacerbations.

Fran is often so exhausted at the end of the day that she has nothing left to offer her husband and children. Fortunately, her children are able to function independently in many ways, but she feels guilty about how little she is able to do for them at this point. Although her husband has been very understanding, she and he are both concerned that her fatigue and inability to participate in shared activities are having an impact on their relationship. She worries that she is not "carrying her weight" in the relationship, and he feels the loss of his much-loved companion and partner. Both are feeling somewhat isolated and alone. Fran asked her family to come to a family counselor with her, to help them get a better understanding of what's happening to her, and provide a structured opportunity for some brainstorming about ways to accommodate her cognitive symptoms and fatigue.

Test Results

Fran's premorbid IQ is estimated in the very superior range. Her language and conceptual reasoning skills continue to be outstanding. Her deficits at this time include problems with verbal memory, divided attention tasks, and shifting between tasks. Her speed of information processing is significantly slowed. Hearing these test results, it began to make sense to Fran why she was having to spend so much more time in the office to get things done, and why she had so little left to give once she was home.

Compensatory Strategies

Fran is working with a cognitive rehabilitation specialist to learn how to minimize the impact of her deficits at home and at work. Together, they have identified a variety of strategies and tools to address the problems she is having. Each evening, Fran plans out the following day in a written schedule, prioritizing her tasks and estimating the amount of time they will take her. Included in that schedule are several five-minute breaks to clear her head, recover her energy, and review her priorities for the remainder of the day.

To help her stay on track during the day, Fran has started jotting down a one-word cue to herself any time she is interrupted in the middle of a task. This helps her remember what she was doing prior to the interruption. When away from office or home (without access to a handy notepad), she carries a hand-held recorder in case she thinks of something she needs to remember to do or write down when she arrives. She also leaves an occasional phone message for herself when she needs to do something as soon as she arrives at the office or home.

Fran is aware that she is going to have to cut back on her workload if she wants to manage at the office and become a more active participant at home. She has already begun to delegate more responsibility to others in the office.

Although it makes her frustrated and sad to think about doing less of the work that she loves, she also recognizes that she is not functioning up to her own standards at work and is missing precious involvement with her husband and sons. Fran is planning to talk with her law partners about working a reduced schedule and specializing in those areas of their general practice in which she excels.

To help keep track of family members' busy schedules, Fran created a shared calendar for the kitchen wall. Each person makes sure that school events, appointments, social activities, sporting events, and travel plans are posted for all to see. This allows Fran to stay in touch with what's going on without having to ask her husband and kids repeatedly what their plans are. The various household chores they all share are also posted on a schedule in the kitchen—this helps everyone remember.

At the suggestion of the rehabilitation specialist, Fran makes the most of her love of games and puzzles. She tries to make time for the daily crossword puzzle in the newspaper and one or two of the game shows on television. These activities have been a relatively fun way to practice her verbal memory skills.

BILL—TAXI DRIVER

Background

Bill, a 33-year-old taxi driver in a small Midwestern city, was diagnosed with MS five years ago. His symptoms include fatigue, mild spasticity in his legs, and optic neuritis that improved after his initial attack. Recently, Bill has been having difficulty remembering the address that his passenger gives him, and he needs to refer repeatedly to the entry in his driver's log. In addition, he finds it harder to navigate around town, because his sense of direction is no longer as good as it used to be. He tends to get distracted if passengers are talking to him or to each other, or the two-way radio is operating. Bill also finds it harder to make quick decisions about a route change if he encounters a detour or traffic jam. His neurologist has encouraged him to start one of the disease-modifying therapies, but he is reluctant because his MS has seemed stable with relatively few physical symptoms. The physician recently pointed out that the medication may slow the progress of his cognitive changes, and Bill is reconsidering his decision.

In the meantime, the doctor has recommended a stretching regimen for the spasticity, as well as an antispasticity medication.

Bill's wife has gotten very anxious about Bill's safety. She doesn't want him to drive a taxi anymore, but is equally anxious about their financial situation and what will happen to them if he has to quit his job. They have two small children, and she is reluctant to start a full-time job until they are older.

Test Results

Bill's premorbid IQ is estimated in the average range. His current deficits, which do not seem to fluctuate very much, include impairments in verbal and visual memory, slowed information processing, difficulty with divided attention tasks, and visual-spatial problems. His language skills, conceptual reasoning, and problem solving appear to be little affected.

Compensatory Strategies

Although he has never had an accident, Bill is very aware that his physical symptoms and cognitive changes could affect his safety and skills as a taxi driver. He knows that he doesn't feel as confident as he used to behind the wheel, and this has made a job that he used to find gratifying much less enjoyable. The company for which he works has been supportive, but his supervisor insisted that he have a driving evaluation to assess his current abilities. His performance on the evaluation was within an acceptable range: His reaction times continue to be adequate, but at the low end of normal, and his overall handling of the car is within the normal range but not as smooth as it once was or as he would like it to be. The evaluation will be repeated in six months to determine if his driving skills are deteriorating or remaining stable.

In the meantime, Bill is utilizing a variety of strategies to help him remain safe and effective on the job. He has taken extra time to "over-learn" the layout of the city by studying neighborhood maps. He wants to be so familiar with the streets that he can remember his way around more easily. He has begun looking into a computerized Global Positioning System (GPS) for the cab in the event that he eventually needs more assistance with directions.

When a passenger gets into the cab and gives the destination, Bill says it aloud while writing it in his log—both of which help him remember it. He also takes a couple of seconds to visualize the route before he starts driving. Bill has also taken to closing the window between the front and back seats so as not to be distracted by conversations with passenger(s). This has been very hard for him since he always enjoyed the social interactions with the people in his cab. He checks in with his dispatcher between customers, but does not leave the radio on while driving.

Bill has scheduled an appointment with a vocational rehabilitation counselor to explore other options in case he becomes unable to continue driving a cab. He has a high school diploma, and hopes that he will be able to train to be a dispatcher if his current job becomes impossible.

SANDRA—MOTHER OF THREE

Background

Sandra is a 35-year-old mother of three children, ages 8, 10, and 14 years. Diagnosed seven years ago, her MS appears to be primary-progressive. Sandra's physician has tried her on a couple of the disease-modifying therapies in hopes of slowing progression, but she has gotten slowly but steadily worse since the diagnosis. She has problems with weakness, poor balance, occasional urinary frequency and urgency, and fatigue, and she uses a cane for mobility.

Sandra finds the hours between 4 PM and 7 PM to be particularly challenging because of the divided attention required for help with homework, dinner preparation, and the chaotic hustle-and-bustle that is inevitable when everyone is at home. On a day-to-day basis, Sandra finds it hard to keep track of the routes when ferrying her children to their various activities, particularly when distracted by their conversations or bickering in the back seat. She even has trouble remembering the activities themselves. She is also finding it increasingly challenging to balance her checkbook; she tends to get confused in the process, losing her train of thought and making calculation errors.

Recently, the children have begun "testing limits" even more than normal. Their own anxieties about the changes they see in their mom are causing them to misbehave and see what they can get away with. Sandra's husband feels overburdened by his own job and the extra responsibilities he has had to take up since her MS has worsened. Sandra's parents, who live in a nearby town, have gotten more involved in an effort to provide support and a helping hand. Although Sandra is grateful for their assistance, it is also one more sign that she cannot handle things the way she used to. She is torn between wanting as much help as they can give, and wanting them to keep their opinions to themselves. She also worries about her ability to be of assistance to them when the time comes that they are not as healthy and independent as they are now.

At one point, Sandra became quite depressed and started on an antidepressant prescribed by her physician. That, in combination with some weekly counseling sessions, has helped considerably.

Test Results

Sandra's estimated premorbid IQ is in the high average range. Her deficits, which remain fairly consistent except when she is very tired or stressed, include impairments in verbal and visual memory, difficulty with divided-attention tasks, problems shifting between tasks, slowed information-processing speed, and visual-spatial problems.

Compensatory Strategies

Sandra is relying on a number of strategies and tools to help her manage the demands of her daily life. At the recommendation of her neurologist, she takes a nap in the afternoon before the kids get home. She has found that this time-out helps her prepare for the busy few hours ahead. Once the children are home, she tries to make sure she has a little time with each one alone—to chat or help with homework in a quiet, distraction-free environment (one of the upstairs bedrooms seems to work best). She has also asked her husband to become more involved with the homework activities. Sandra keeps a family calendar, with each child's after-school activities posted clearly. Each evening, she writes out her schedule for the next day, including how much time she estimates that each activity will take. She carries the schedule with her and makes a note of how long each activity actually takes. This comparison helps her plan more accurately on subsequent days.

Sandra consulted with a cognitive rehabilitation specialist about ways to make her household tasks more manageable. She started by designating a spot in the kitchen for her sunglasses, keys, and wallet, to cut down on the amount of time spent looking for things. She has started using a checkbook with duplicate checks to minimize errors when she balances the account, and has asked her husband to check it over for errors. Although her husband has offered to take over the banking activities, Sandra has always taken pride in her ability to handle this aspect of their lives and wants to continue as long as she can.

Sandra designated a spot for all the mail that comes in and bought a filing rack for her desk, in which each hanging folder is stamped with a day of the month. When she opens a bill, she puts it in the folder indicating the date when she needs to mail payment. This ensures that the mail doesn't get lost and that the bills are paid in a timely fashion. Sandra has already been able to cut down significantly on late fees.

With the help of the rehabilitation specialist, Sandra created a series of templates. First, she created seven basic meal plans. These help her track the necessary ingredients and preparation plans all in one place and simplify her shopping as well. To make shopping even easier, she uses a master grocery list (that her 14-year-old helped create on the computer and prints out for her on a weekly basis) that enables her to review the list and check off the items she needs to buy each week rather than having to think up the list from scratch each time. In other words, the master list acts as a series of cues to help her remember the things she might need. Sandra has a white board on the wall in the kitchen to jot down the grocery items she has run out of; this assists her in filling out the weekly shopping list.

Sandra also created a file of directions to carry with her in the car for those trips she makes on a routine basis—for example, the route to and from soccer practice, playmates' houses, particular stores. While she doesn't need to refer to the templates very often, it reassures her to know that they are there in the car with her.

At the suggestion of the rehabilitation specialist, the family sits down periodically to review the current strategies and brainstorm new ones. These family meetings have helped immensely: They ensure that Sandra's husband and children have a better sense of what's going on and what they and Sandra can do to keep things running smoothly; Sandra feels less alone and less stressed; and the children feel reassured that everything is, and will continue to be, managed.

Sandra has also been working on some stress management techniques of her own to help her feel better. The family meets periodically with a family therapist to help them talk with one another about the MS-related changes in their lives.

JEFF—CONSTRUCTION WORKER

Background

Jeff is a 37-year-old construction worker employed by a company that specializes in the construction of shopping centers. He and his wife have been married for 10 years, and he has two small children. Jeff was diagnosed with MS five years ago, following an episode of optic neuritis and numbness in his hands. He had his first attack of optic neuritis at age 17, but the diagnosis could not be confirmed at that time. Although the optic neuritis cleared, Jeff still has mild sensory loss in his hands and feet, and has developed spasticity, fatigue, erectile problems, and bladder and bowel problems that are managed with medications. He has found that his symptoms feel much worse when he becomes overheated. Jeff started on a disease-modifying therapy about six months following the diagnosis.

Jeff is having increasing difficulty on the job. He finds that tools will at times slip from his grasp due to his sensory problems, especially when he is overheated. He has also been misjudging distances and gets distracted from the task at hand by other things going on around him. In addition, he is finding it difficult to understand the concepts behind construction drawings, follow them accurately, and translate them into action. His wife has noticed that he has problems doing things around the house that used to be easy for him. She is concerned and confused, and unsure what it all means. She finds herself getting very angry at him for not being as helpful as he used to be, but then feels guilty about it. She stopped working when her first child was born, with the hope of being a full-time mom until both kids reached high-school age. Worries about his wife and children, and his ability to support them, have added significantly to Jeff's stress.

Test Results

Jeff's estimated premorbid IQ is in the average range. He graduated in the middle of his class in high school but always had particular skill with his hands. His language skills and memory remain intact at this time. Current deficits include impairments in divided attention, conceptual reasoning, and visual-spatial organization—difficult challenges for someone who works in a busy construction site. His information-processing speed has slowed considerably.

Compensatory Strategies

Jeff knows that he has had a number of near misses that could have affected his safety and the safety of others, but only recently has he discussed his problems with his foreman. He had not previously disclosed his MS because he had no visible symptoms, but finally decided he needed to let them know that he has MS and that cognitive changes are one way in which MS can affect a person. Jeff is going to request assignment to particular jobs in the shopping mall that are less complex and more repetitive. He will also explore ways to create a less distracting environment, such as wearing earplugs or working in a more isolated corner of the job. At the recommendation of his neurologist, Jeff now wears a cooling vest at all times to help maintain his core body temperature. He has already discovered that his sensory symptoms are less of a problem.

Jeff and his doctor have discussed the possibility that he may soon need to leave construction work, particularly if he cannot arrange for different types of projects. Although Jeff's foreman hasn't said anything yet, Jeff is aware that he and the other crew members are starting to get uncomfortable. They watch him more than they used to, and Jeff is certain that they are increasingly concerned about his safety as well as their own. The members of a construction team need to be able to count on one another if the job is going to get done safely and well. The doctor referred Jeff to vocational rehabilitation to explore other job possibilities, such as office work in a construction company, doing light repair work, or changing his field all together.

Jeff and his wife have begun to discuss the possibility of her returning to work, at least on a part-time basis, so that they will be more prepared in the event that he becomes unable to work full-time. This discussion has been very stressful for both of them, and they are thinking of asking their National Multiple Sclerosis Society chapter for a referral to a family therapist who could help them talk about their options more comfortably.

STAN—RETIRED SECURITIES ANALYST

Background

Stan is a 50-year-old former securities analyst. He developed primary-progressive MS at the age of 34 and had to retire on disability nine years ago, when his fatigue, balance problems, weakness, and bladder dysfunction made it impossible for him to work a full day and do the necessary business travel. He now uses a manual wheelchair outside the house and a walker at home. He is divorced and lives alone.

Although Stan had experienced some cognitive changes prior to retirement, they were not serious enough to keep him from performing the duties of his job. Within the last several years, however, Stan's cognitive problems have gotten significantly worse. He has trouble remembering what he has to do when, where he put his glasses or keys, or where to find things in his house. He is also finding it harder to keep track of his medications and generally take care of himself. Planning and preparing meals are a major challenge. When driving, Stan finds that his reaction times feel "sticky," and that he gets lost easily and is often distracted by things going on around him. He has been driving adequately with the hand controls that were recommended during an initial driving evaluation, but no longer feels as confident—and his friends are no longer willing to ride with him. Stan has increasing difficult remembering faces and names, and does not always remember to call people back. All these problems have led to some misunderstandings and increased social isolation.

Stan used to pride himself on doing his own taxes, but can no longer deal with all of the IRS rules and regulations. Once an avid reader, he finds it hard now to follow a story and remember the characters or track the main points of a newspaper or magazine article. Stan's neurologist recently referred him to a psychiatrist for an evaluation to determine if depression might be contributing to his cognitive problems. He was put on an antidepressant that provided some relief but did not significantly improve his cognitive functioning.

Test Results

Stan's premorbid IQ is estimated to have been in the high superior range. Currently, his deficits include impairments in verbal and visual memory and conceptual reasoning, as well as slowed information-processing speed and problems with visual tracking. The tests also showed that Stan tires easily on any task that requires prolonged concentration. Seeing these results helped Stan understand why he has been having so much difficulty with his daily activities. Although it was painful to see the evidence of his deficits, he also found the information helpful because it enabled him to begin thinking about how he might begin to deal with them in a constructive way. A problem-solver by nature, Stan began to use his "smarts" to find ways around the problems.

Compensatory Strategies

Stan's neurologist has referred him for another driving evaluation. In the meantime, the doctor has also filled out an application to the state paratransit system so that Stan will have the ability to get to daytime appointments and activities. Because the public system does not run after 7 PM, Stan is planning to enlist help from his friends to get to social activities. In the process of discussing this with his friends, Stan will try to help them understand more about his cognitive symptoms, in hopes of reducing some of the recent strain in their relationships and getting him re-involved in a social life.

With the help of a cognitive remediation specialist, Stan has developed some strategies to help make reading enjoyable again. He highlights points in the text that he wants to be able to refer back to, and keeps a running list of characters and main events on an index card. He places the index card under each line as he is reading, which makes it easier for him to concentrate and significantly lessens his fatigue. To avoid losing the index card, he also uses it as a bookmark. Although these strategies haven't enabled him to read at the pace he once used to, they have made it possible for him to enjoy and remember what he does choose to read.

The remediation specialist worked with Stan to create several simple but nourishing meal plans. These have helped Stan with his shopping list and given him a bit more confidence about his ability to get a meal on the table; he's even thinking about inviting some friends to join him for dinner occasionally. Stan and the specialist created a shopping template that follows the aisles in his neighborhood store. This allows Stan to avoid going through the whole store; he only needs to visit those aisles in which items he needs are located.

Stan is also working with the remediation specialist on ways to make better use of his computer. He is learning to use it to organize his appointments and maintain all his lists and reminders. When one of his physicians has added or changed a medication, he updates the list so that he always has a current summary of his medications to share with his health care providers. He is also capitalizing on his enjoyment of computer games to try and improve his concentration. Stan recently purchased computerized versions of a couple of TV game shows to exercise his verbal memory abilities.

At his neurologist's suggestion, Stan brings a tape recorder to every appointment so that he can review what they talked about when he's back home. He also bought himself a watch with multiple alarms to help him remember when to take his medications.

With the help of an organization consultant, he is gradually rear-ranging things in his house so that everything has a specific place. This will make it easier for him to remember from one time to another where things are supposed to be so that he won't have to spend so much time hunting. He has also posted a list by the door of the things he needs to have with him whenever he goes out—wallet, keys, and other necessities.

Stan is hoping that these various strategies will help him to remain active and independent. He knows that being inactive and isolated makes his depression worse. If his cognitive symptoms continue to progress, he will consider transitioning to some kind of assistive-living facility, so that he can get the assistance he needs while remaining as active and socially involved as he wants to be.

KENDRA—EXECUTIVE

Background

Kendra is a 56-year-old executive in an insurance company. Her children are grown, and she lives at home with her husband. She was diagnosed with MS 20 years ago. Her symptoms, which are mostly invisible to others, include fatigue; sensory changes in her hands and feet; bladder, bowel, and sexual dysfunction; and occasional problems with blurred vision.

Kendra finds that she can still do the things that she used to do but not as quickly or as efficiently as before. Her ability to analyze complex business plans is not what it used to be, and she has lost confidence in her ability to take on and successfully complete large projects. Kendra has trouble remembering the names of new business contacts and keeping track of her appointments and meetings. Fortunately, she has a secretary who manages her schedule, answers her phone, and maintains a list of people she needs to call. Each day, the secretary prints out Kendra's schedule and phone call list so that Kendra has them with her at all times. Kendra knows that without that assistance, she would be having a great deal of difficulty managing her daily activities.

Kendra is menopausal, and recent mood swings may be the result of either hormone changes or the MS. She consulted a psychiatrist about her mood swings and was told that she could start on some medication if they become too uncomfortable. Kendra knows from her friends of a similar age that many of them are also experiencing some problems with memory and thinking. This has made it difficult for Kendra to figure out how much of her difficulty is related to age and menopause, and how much to MS, particularly since her friends are always telling her not to worry—"we're all just getting older."

Without a secretary at home to help her, Kendra is having difficult staying connected with people and activities. She does not remember to return calls, which has led to quite a few misunderstandings.

Kendra's husband works in advertising. He is trying to be supportive, but has difficulty understanding and accepting the cognitive changes he sees in his wife. Having always been attracted to her quick and agile mind, he is having far more difficulty dealing with her cognitive symptoms than with her physical ones. He has a tendency to get irritated with her, convinced that if she just "tried harder," she could manage things better.

Test Results

Kendra's premorbid IQ is estimated to have been in the superior range. Fortunately, she has always been a highly organized and efficient person, and will be able to use those abilities to help compensate for the cognitive changes she is experiencing.

Over the past few years, Kendra's deficits have generally been stable or very slowly progressive, but she has noticed a slow, downward trend since she entered the perimenopausal period. Her problems now include mild impairments in attention, conceptual reasoning, verbal memory, and planning and prioritizing, as well as slowed information processing. Her visual memory has been relatively unaffected.

Compensatory Strategies

With the help of a cognitive remediation specialist, Kendra is learning to substitute organization for memory wherever possible. In addition to the help provided by her secretary, Kendra is learning to make optimal use of her electronic organizer, her computer, and filing systems at work and at home. She is learning to utilize her strong visual memory skills to compensate for the verbal memory impairment, including taking notes during meetings and conversations; posting reminders for herself in the office and at home; using visual cues to help her remember names; and utilizing a master grocery list—organized according to the layout of the store—to plan her weekly purchases.

To assist with her projects at work, Kendra is looking into various kinds of project planning and management software to help her plan and organize her work. She is also working on some simple analysis templates to help her think through various types of decisions in a more focused, systematic fashion. The templates help her identify the major issues involved, as well as the various pros and cons for each decision.

In the meantime, Kendra is talking with her cognitive remediation specialist about strategies for alleviating pressure at work, as well as options for the future should she need to transition from her current position to a slower one with less pressure. She and the specialist are meeting on a regular basis to ensure that she is making maximum use of compensatory strategies.

At the suggestion of the remediation specialist, Kendra asked her husband to attend a couple of remediation sessions with her. The neuropsychologist reviewed Kendra's test findings with both of them, taking the time to explain to Kendra's husband more about the changes she has been experiencing and answer his questions. Kendra realized that, in her efforts to shield her husband from what was going on, she hadn't taken the time to help him understand her problems, or to involve him in her compensatory strategies. This has helped to revive the strong feelings of partnership that the two had shared earlier in their relationship.

ELIZABETH—ELEMENTARY SCHOOL LEARNING SPECIALIST

Background

Elizabeth is a 45-year-old learning specialist who was diagnosed with MS at age 35. She is divorced, and has one son who is away at college. Initially diagnosed with relapsing-remitting disease, Elizabeth has been on a disease-modifying medication for the past eight years. Her physician has recently told her that her MS is now secondary-progressive, and they are considering a change in her treatment. She deals with her primary symptoms of fatigue and leg weakness by using a cane for short distances and a motorized scooter for longer ones. She manages her bladder symptoms with medication and intermittent self-catheterization.

Elizabeth's job requires that she travel between three elementary schools in the district, meeting on a regular basis with small groups of children who are in need of remedial help. Until fairly recently, she has managed the complexities of the job very well, using her accessible van to get from one location to another. The school system has provided accommodations in the form of a convenient parking space at each of the schools and air-conditioned offices that are close to the bathroom.

Recently, however, Elizabeth has been finding it increasingly difficult to coordinate her complex schedule, keep track of her many students, and organize her student records and teaching materials— much of which she has to carry around with her from school to school. Her fatigue, which is significant by the middle of the day, has begun to impact her ability to think clearly, focus on what she is trying to do, and make the best use of the time with her students. Because her teaching is so individualized, she needs constantly to be evaluating each student's progress and planning accordingly for the next session. Elizabeth's supervisor, who has always been supportive of her teaching efforts and responsive to her requests for accommodations, has begun to express impatience and frustration with her recent disorganization and tardiness with reports.

Test Results

Elizabeth's premorbid intelligence is estimated in the high average to superior range. Although her verbal and visual memory scores remain within normal limits, they probably reflect a significant decrease, given Elizabeth's academic background. She appears to have experienced a similar decline in information-processing speed and executive functions, as reflected in her problems with planning, organization, and report writing. Elizabeth's performance during her neuropsychological evaluation provided clear evidence that fatigue significantly impacts her cognitive abilities over the course of the day and confirmed that pacing in her daily schedule is essential.

Compensatory Strategies

As a single woman with a college-age child, Elizabeth is highly concerned about her ability to continue in her profession. She needs and loves her job with the school system—not only as a source of personal satisfaction and self-esteem, but also for the financial security and health insurance benefits it provides. Via referrals from her National Multiple Sclerosis Society chapter, Elizabeth has sought the advice of both an employment counselor and a cognitive remediation specialist to help her identify her options.

Elizabeth discussed with the employment counselor her concerns about requesting further accommodations from the school.

Although her supervisor had been supportive of her requests in the past, Elizabeth was worried that additional requests—this time for problems that are cognitive rather than physical—would not get a very good response. The employment counselor assured her that accommodations for cognitive symptoms were just as valid a request as any other, and that her strategy with her supervisor should be to explain how the requested strategies would enhance her organization, productivity, and outcomes on the job.

Together, Elizabeth and the counselor developed a list of requested accommodations: a schedule that would allow her to work in only one school per day; an office space in each school that would accommodate her student files and a complete set of educational materials, to eliminate the need to carry them around with her; and a flexible schedule to allow for brief rest periods throughout the course of the day. The counselor offered to meet with Elizabeth and the supervisor if the need arose.

With the help of the cognitive remediation specialist, Elizabeth developed several strategies to help her conserve energy and organize her schedule and tasks more effectively. They created a report-writing template to make the process easier and more efficient. This not only helped with the reports themselves, but also made it easier for Elizabeth to remember what was going on with each child from week to week. The specialist suggested a filing system for the office that made it easier for Elizabeth to keep track of her educational materials and records, and an office arrangement that allowed her to reach most of her files without getting up from her chair. Together, they figured out how frequently Elizabeth needed to take breaks to minimize the impact of her fatigue on her cognitive skills. At the specialist's suggestion, Elizabeth created flash cards to help her remember her students' names and the main focus of their remedial work.

The supervisor responded positively to the coherent plan that Elizabeth proposed. By explaining the accommodations clearly—with some input from both the employment counselor and the remediation specialist—Elizabeth was able to convince her supervisor that, at least for the time being, she would be able to provide quality care for her students. The supervisor said he would make every effort to have Elizabeth go to only one school per day during the coming school year, assuming that the students' schedules could be arranged accordingly. He agreed to the other accommodations as well, with the stipulation that Elizabeth needed to be able to fulfill her teaching responsibilities successfully to keep her position. If, in periodic reviews, it was determined that she was unable to fulfill those responsibilities adequately, she would not be able to stay in the position.

Although Elizabeth now feels more confident about her ability to continue in her job, she is also working with the vocational counselor to identify possible options in the event that she becomes unable to continue in her current position with the school system.

CONCLUSIONS

Obviously, no series of vignettes can cover all the circumstances that people with MS encounter in their daily lives. Our goal has been to put the MS-related cognitive changes into real-life settings so that you and your family members and friends can visualize the various ways in which a person might be impacted by these changes and the strategies that can help make these changes more manageable. You may find as you read these vignettes that you can develop a similar portrait of your own situation. Stepping back in this way—perhaps to take a more objective view of your activities at home and at work—may help you pinpoint some of the changes you have experienced and identify some adaptations or changes that would work for you. Keep in mind, however, that there is no need to go through this process alone. A variety of resources are available to help you along the way.

PROFESSIONAL BIOGRAPHIES

OF THE AUTHORS

LAUREN CARUSO, PhD

Lauren Caruso is a neuropsychologist who has specialized in cognitive difficulties in persons with MS for over 18 years. At the Medication Rehabilitation Research and Training Center for MS at Albert Einstein College of Medicine and subsequently at St. Agnes Hospital/New York Medical College, Dr. Caruso worked with Drs. LaRocca and Kalb on a number of innovative research projects focused on cognitive changes in MS.

Dr. Caruso is currently the director of the Cognitive Division of the Multiple Sclerosis Research Center of New York, in New York City. In addition, she sees patients at the Multiple Sclerosis Center at White Plains Hospital in White Plains, New York and in private practice. She provides neuropsychological evaluations for children, young adults, and the elderly, as well as providing individually tailored cognitive remediation. Dr. Caruso is Clinical Assistant Professor of Neurology and Psychiatry at New York Medical College and is licensed as a psychologist in New York.

Dr. Caruso serves on the Clinical Advisory Committees of the Southern New York and New York City Chapters of the National Multiple Sclerosis Society. She has given numerous workshops and lectures on cognition for lay and professional audiences.

JOHN DeLUCA, PhD

John DeLuca is director of Neuroscience Research at the Kessler Medical Rehabilitation Research and Education Corporation (KMRREC) and a professor in the Departments of Physical Medicine & Rehabilitation (PM&R) and Neurosciences at University of Medicine and Dentistry of New Jersey-New Jersey Medical School (UMDNJ-NJMS), where he also directs the post-doctoral fellowship program in neuropsychology. He is licensed as a psychologist in the States of New Jersey and New York. Dr. DeLuca is currently studying disorders of memory and information processing in a variety of clinical populations including multiple sclerosis, traumatic brain injury, and chronic fatigue syndrome patients.

Dr. DeLuca has published over 200 scientific articles, abstracts, and chapters. His most recent book is entitled *Fatigue as a Window to the Brain*. He is an associate editor of the *Archives of Physical Medicine and Rehabilitation* and serves on the editorial board of several other prominent journals. Dr. DeLuca is the recipient of early career awards for his research from both the American Psychological Association and the National Academy of Neuropsychology, and he received the Distinguished Researcher Award in 2005 from the New Jersey Psychological Association. He is also a Fellow of the American Psychological Association and the National Academy of Neuropsychology. Dr. DeLuca has received numerous federal and private grants, and currently is the principal investigator or co-investigator on three active federal grants and a consultant to two others. He has served on the board of trustees for New York Neuropsychology Group and the New Jersey Neuropsychological Society, and as president of this latter organization.

ROSALIND KALB, PhD

Rosalind Kalb, a clinical psychologist, is director of the Professional Resource Center at the National Multiple Sclerosis Society in New York City, where she develops and provides educational materials and consultation services for health care professionals. Dr. Kalb began her career in MS providing individual, group, and family therapy at the MS Care Center at the Albert Einstein College of Medicine. Following the Center's relocation to New York Medical College, Dr. Kalb added a variety of other clinical and research activities to her work in MS, including groups for well spouses and couples living with MS, and neuropsychological evaluation and cognitive rehabilitation for research and treatment purposes. In her private practice, over the past 25 years, Dr. Kalb has provided individual, group, and family therapy for people living with MS.

Dr. Kalb has authored or edited a number of publications about multiple sclerosis. She is the author of *Families Affected by Multiple Sclerosis: Disease Impacts and Coping Strategies*, a monograph published in 1995 by the National Multiple Sclerosis Society and of the

Society's *Knowledge Is Power* series for individuals newly diagnosed with MS. She is also the editor of the Society's booklet series for health professionals entitled *Talking with Your MS Patients about Difficult Topics*, and serves on the editorial board of *Keep S'myelin*, the newsletter for children who have a parent with MS. Dr. Kalb has edited two books—*Multiple Sclerosis: The Questions You Have, The Answers You Need*, published in its third edition in 2004, and *Multiple Sclerosis: A Guide for Families*, published in its third edition in 2006.

NICHOLAS LaROCCA, PhD

Nicholas LaRocca, a clinical psychologist who has worked in the field of MS for over 27 years, is director of Health Care Delivery and Policy Research at the National Multiple Sclerosis Society in New York. In this role, he directs programs that fund MS research in symptomatic management, rehabilitation, quality of life, psychosocial issues, and health policy.

Before coming to work for the National Multiple Sclerosis Society, Dr. LaRocca was the director of research at the Medical Rehabilitation Research and Training Center (RTC) for MS at Albert Einstein College of Medicine and then at St. Agnes Hospital/New York Medical College, where he was associate professor of Neurology and Medicine. At the RTC, Dr. LaRocca did extensive clinical work and research focused on the psychosocial and cognitive aspects of MS. He was one of a small group of clinicians and researchers who worked to win greater recognition for the psychological impact of MS, particularly cognitive changes.

Dr. LaRocca has led support groups for persons with MS and their spouses and has given innumerable workshops and presentations for both lay and professional audiences, particularly in the area of cognition. His research interests include assessment methods, psychological issues, cognitive rehabilitation, and quality of life. He is the author of a number of scientific papers and book chapters, and serves on the editorial boards of *The Journal of Rehabilitation Research & Development* and *Real Living with MS*.

GLOSSARY

Activities of daily living (ADLs): Skills necessary for independent living. *Instrumental ADLs* include the ability to use the telephone, shop, cook, perform housekeeping tasks, manage finances, take medications reliably. *Personal ADLs* include toileting, eating, dressing, grooming, bathing.

Alternate test forms. Versions of a cognitive test that are constructed to be identical in format and similar in content. They have also have been shown to be consistent and reliable in measuring the same cognitive function(s), so that they can be used interchangeably.

Anterograde memory. The ability to remember information acquired after disease onset or a brain injury; often differentiated from retrograde memory. *See* Retrograde memory.

Acquisition phase (of memory process). The phase of the memory process in which information is gathered via sensory input, and then processed and organized for storage in the brain. Also commonly referred to as "encoding" or "learning."

Attention. Processes that enable a person to: (a) focus and maintain interest in a given task or activity, often referred to as *sustained attention*; (b) engage in certain cognitive operations while ignoring others (i.e., a selective awareness of or responsiveness to internal or external stimuli), often referred to as *selective attention*; (c) alternate between two or more tasks or activities, often referred to as *alternating attention*.

Autonomic nervous system (ANS). The part of the nervous system that regulates involuntary vital functions, including the activity of the cardiac (heart) muscle, smooth muscles (e.g., of the gut), and glands. The ANS has two divisions. the sympathetic nervous system that accelerates heart rate, constricts blood vessels, and raises blood pressure; the parasympathetic nervous system that slows heart rate, increases intestinal and gland activity, and relaxes sphincter muscles.

Central nervous system (CNS). The part of the nervous system that contains the brain and spinal cord, including the cranial nerves (e.g. the optic nerves).

Cerebellum. A large structure located in the lower posterior region of the brain, which integrates sensory perception and motor output and plays an important role in balance and the coordination of movement.

Cerebral atrophy. The shrinkage of brain tissue that seems to be due, at least in part, to the destruction of myelin and axons. This shrinkage occurs gradually as part of the normal aging process, and more rapidly in connection with certain diseases. In MS, atrophy has been shown to occur even in the earliest stages of the disease.

Cerebrum. The largest and most developed part of the brain, which acts as a master control system and is responsible for initiating thought and motor activity. Its two hemispheres, united by the corpus callosum, form the largest part of the central nervous system.

Chunking. The process of reorganizing materials in working memory in order to increase the number of items successfully recalled. It is easier, for example to remember a series of eight numbers if one breaks the list of eight into four groups of two (39-41-65-27 rather than 39416527). *See* Working memory.

Cognition. The highest-level functions carried out by the human brain, including comprehension and use of speech, visual perception and construction, calculation ability, attention (information processing), memory, and executive functions such as planning, problem-solving, and self-monitoring. *See* Attention; Executive functions.

Cognitive impairment. Declines in cognitive function caused by brain injury or disease process. Some degree of cognitive impairment occurs in approximately one-half to two-thirds of people with MS, with memory, information processing, and executive functions being the most commonly affected functions. *See* Memory; Executive functions.

Cognitive rehabilitation. Techniques designed to improve the functioning of individuals whose cognition is impaired because of brain injury or disease. Rehabilitation strategies are designed to improve the impaired function via repetitive drills and practice or compensatory strategies designed to circumvent impaired functions that are not likely to improve. Cognitive rehabilitation is provided by psychologists, neuropsychologists, speech/language pathologists, and occupational therapists. Although these specialists use different assessment tools and treatment strategies, they share the common goal of improving the individual's ability to function as independently and safely as possible in the home and work environment. *See* Compensatory strategy; Neuropsychologist; Occupational therapist; Speech/language pathologist.

Compensatory strategy. An alternative method of performing a task that substitutes a new way of doing things for an old way that is no longer feasible or possible because of impairment or disability. For example, a person with memory impairment may utilize a paper or electronic calendar to track daily tasks/appointments.

Cued recall. Memory recall in which information about items to be recalled is provided. Common cues include category (e.g., animals, fruits, etc.) and first letter (e.g., words beginning with "t").

Declarative memory. The aspect of memory that stores facts and events, such as standard textbook learning and knowledge. It is also commonly referred to as *explicit memory*. Declarative memory and procedural memory comprise what we think of as memory. Declarative memory can be further divided into *episodic memory* and *semantic memory*. *See* Episodic memory; Procedural memory; Semantic memory.

Dementia. A generalized loss of cognitive functions—which must include memory loss—resulting from a brain injury or disease and negatively impacting social or vocational functioning. The loss, depending on the underlying cause, may progress rapidly or slowly.

Depression. A mood disturbance—characterized by pervasive sadness, loss of pleasure or interest in everyday things, and a general slowing of physical and emotional responses—which persists for at least two weeks. The symptoms of depression include:

- Persistent sad, anxious, or "empty" mood
- Feelings of hopelessness, pessimism
- Feelings of guilt, worthlessness, helplessness
- Loss of interest or pleasure in hobbies and activities that were once enjoyed, including sex
- Decreased energy, fatigue, being "slowed down"*
- Difficulty concentrating, remembering, making decisions*

- Insomnia, early-morning awakening, or oversleeping*
- Appetite and/or weight loss or overeating and weight gain
- Thoughts of death or suicide; suicide attempts
- Restlessness, irritability
- Persistent physical symptoms that do not respond to treatment, such as headaches, digestive disorders, and chronic pain*

The diagnosis of depression in a person with MS can be complicated by the fact that some of the symptoms on this list (those marked with *) are common in both illnesses.

Disability. As defined by the World Health Organization, a disability (resulting from an impairment) is a restriction or lack of ability to perform an activity in the manner or within the range considered normal for a human being.

Disease course. The natural progression of an illness or condition. MS tends to take one of four clinical courses, each of which might be mild, moderate, or severe:

- **Relapsing-remitting MS (RRMS).** The most common form of MS, characterized by partial or total recovery after attacks (also called exacerbations, relapses, or flares). Approximately 75%–85% of people with MS initially begin with a relapsing-remitting course.
- **Secondary-progressive MS (SPMS).** A clinical course of MS that begins as relapsing-remitting (with partial or total recovery after attacks) and subsequently becomes progressive at a variable rate. Attacks and partial recoveries may continue to occur, but with progression in between. Of those who start with relapsing-remitting disease, most will eventually transition to a secondary-progressive course.
- **Primary-progressive MS (PPMS).** A progressive course from onset without any attacks. The symptoms that occur along the way generally do not remit. Ten percent of people with MS are diagnosed with PPMS, although the diagnosis usually needs to be made after the fact—when the person has been living for a period of time with progressive disability but no acute attacks.
- **Progressive-relapsing MS (PRMS).** The rarest disease course in MS (approximately 5% of people), characterized by disease progression from onset, with obvious, acute attacks along the way.

Divided attention. The ability to focus on more than one stimulus or activity at a time.

Episodic memory. The memory for events—including time, place, and associated emotions (e.g., the name of your second- grade teacher, your first date, your wedding anniversary). It is most often contrasted with *semantic memory*, which refers to the recall of facts and concepts that are not tied to specific time or place of learning. Episodic memory is more easily impaired than semantic memory, perhaps because there tends to be less rehearsal or repetition. Episodic and semantic memory together form what is known as *declarative memory*. *See* Declarative memory; Semantic memory.

Evoked potentials (EPs). Recordings of the nervous system's electrical response to the stimulation of specific sensory pathways (e.g., visual, auditory, general sensory). In tests of evoked potentials, a person's recorded responses are displayed on an oscilloscope and analyzed on a computer that allows comparison with normal response times. Demyelination results in a slowing of response time. EPs can demonstrate lesions along specific nerve pathways, whether or not the lesions are producing symptoms or not, thus making this test useful in confirming the diagnosis of MS. Visual evoked potentials are considered the most useful in MS.

Executive functions. Cognitive abilities that are required for complex, goal-oriented behaviors, including initiating, planning, prioritizing, sequencing, goal-setting, decision-making, self-monitoring, self-correcting, and the organization and execution of multi-step tasks.

Expanded Disability Status Scale (EDSS). A part of the Minimal Record of Disability that summarizes the neurologic examination and provides a measure of overall disability. The EDSS is a 20-point scale, ranging from 0 (normal examination) to 10 (death due to MS) by half-points. A person with a score of 4.5 can walk three blocks without stopping; a score of 6.0 means that a cane or a leg brace is needed to walk one block; a score over 7.5 indicates that a person cannot take more than a few steps, even with crutches or help from another person. The EDSS is used for many reasons, including deciding future medical treatment, establishing rehabilitation goals, choosing subjects for participation in clinical trials, and measuring treatment outcomes. This is currently the most widely used scale in clinical trials.

Free recall. The ability to retrieve something from memory (e.g., a word, fact, or name) without any external cues or prompts.

Frontal lobe. The largest portion of each cerebral hemisphere, lying directly behind the forehead and considered to be the most highly evolved area of the brain. The frontal lobes are involved in motor function, expressive language, executive functions, problem-solving and reasoning, spontaneity, acquisition, judgment, impulse control, and social and sexual behavior. The frontal lobes assist in planning, coordinating, controlling, and carrying out actions. *See* Executive functions.

Full-Scale IQ. A measure of general intellectual functioning. On intelligence tests like the Wechsler Adult Intelligence Scale, the Full Scale IQ score is a composite of the subtest scores on the Verbal and Performance components of the test.

Functional MRI (fMRI). A technique for determining which parts of the brain are activated by different types of physical sensation or activity, such as sight, sound, or the movement of a subject's fingers. This "brain mapping" is achieved by setting up an advanced MRI scanner in a special way so that the increased blood flow to the activated areas of the brain shows up on fMRI scans.

Hypothalamic-pituitary-adrenal (HPA) axis. A major part of the neuroendocrine system that controls reactions to stress and plays an important role in regulating various bodily functions, such as digestion, the immune system, and energy usage. The HPA axis enables a set of interactions among glands, hormones, and parts of the midbrain that constitute the body's general adaptation response to stress.

Immune system. A complex network of glands, tissues, circulating cells, and processes that protect the body by identifying abnormal or foreign substances and neutralizing them.

Impairment. As defined by the World Health Organization, an impairment is any loss or abnormality of psychological, physiological, or anatomical structure or function. It represents a deviation from the person's usual biomedical state. An impairment is thus any loss of function directly resulting from injury or disease.

Intelligence. A concept that refers to the ability to understand complex ideas, adapt effectively to the environment, learn from experience, engage in various types of thinking and reasoning, and overcome obstacles by thinking, planning, problem-solving.

Lesion. An area of damaged tissue resulting from disease or trauma. In MS, the term refers to an area of inflamed or demyelinated central nervous system tissue (also called a *"plaque"*). The multiple areas of scarring created by lesions in the CNS are what give multiple sclerosis its name.

Long-term memory. The retention of any information that has been considered sufficiently important to be stored in the brain "indefinitely" for later retrieval (e.g., what you had for dinner last night, the headline in today's paper, what your boss told you this morning about your request for a job transfer).

Magnetic resonance imaging (MRI). A diagnostic procedure that produces visual images of different body parts without the use of X-rays. Nuclei of atoms are influenced by a high-frequency electromagnetic impulse inside a strong magnetic field. The nuclei then give off resonating signals that can produce pictures of parts of the body. An important diagnostic tool in MS, MRI makes it possible to visualize and count lesions in the white matter of the brain and spinal cord.

Memory. The acquisition and retention of information. A variety of terms have been used to classify different memory functions. *See* Anterograde memory; Declarative memory; Episodic memory; Long-term memory; Procedural memory; Retrograde memory; Semantic memory; Working memory.

Mental status examination. A method (including both observation and interview) of evaluating orientation (name, date, place), attention and concentration, memory, language, visual-spatial skills, insight, abstraction, general cognitive function, and/or psychiatric status. The "bedside (or physician's office) mental status examination" may include some or all of these areas. The standard examination that is incorporated into the neurologic examination is fairly global and insensitive to early cognitive change; it has been shown to miss approximately 50% of people with MS-related cognitive impairment.

MRI. *See* Magnetic resonance imaging.

Neuropsychologist (clinical neuropsychologist). A psychologist with special training and expertise in the applied science of brain-behavior relationships. Clinical neuropsychologists use this knowledge in the assessment, diagnosis, treatment, and/or rehabilitation of patients across the lifespan with neurologic or other medical conditions, as well as cognitive and learning disorders. The clinical neuro-psychologist uses psychological, neurologic, cognitive, behavioral, and physiological principles, techniques, and tests to evaluate a person's cognitive strengths and weaknesses and their relationship to normal and abnormal central nervous system functioning. The clinical neuropsychologist uses this information, and information provided by other medical/health care providers, to identify and diagnose cognitive changes or problems, and plan and implement intervention strategies.

Occupational therapist (OT). A health care professional who assesses functioning in those activities of daily living—including dressing, bathing, grooming, meal preparation, writing, and driving—which that are essential for independent living. In making treatment recommendations, the OT addresses (a) fatigue management; (b) upper body strength, movement, and coordination; (c) adaptations to the home and work environment, including both structural changes and specialized equipment for particular activities; and (d) compensatory strategies for impairments in thinking, sensation, or vision.

Percentile. A score indicating the percentage of scores at or below the comparison value (e.g., an individual who scores in the 85% percentile on a given test has performed better than 85% percent of those taking the test).

Performance IQ. A composite score that summarizes the Performance scale subtest scores obtained on a test battery measuring intellectual abilities (e.g., the Wechsler Adult Intelligence Scale [WAIS]). It is commonly considered a measure of non-verbal cognitive functioning and may also be used to derive premorbid estimates. *See* Premorbid estimation.

PET. *See* Positron emission tomography.

Positron emission tomography. A computerized radiographic technique that uses radioactive substances for imaging metabolic or physiological functions in different parts of the body, including the brain. The person either inhales or is injected with a biochemical that carries a radioactive substance. This substance sends out positively-charged particles (positrons) that combine with the negatively-charged electrons normally found in cells of the body. The combination of positrons and electrons produces gamma rays that are detected by the PET device and converted into color-coded images. The images indicate the intensity of the metabolic activity of the organ being studied.

Practice effects. Improvements in test performance as a result of having taken the test previously. Practice effects generally increase with each additional exposure to the test items.

Premorbid estimation. Methods of estimating a person's level of cognitive ability prior to injury or the onset of illness. Premorbid estimates are most commonly derived from those aspects of current test performance that are least likely to be affected by brain injury or disease (e.g., reading decoding skills and vocabulary), taking into account the individual's academic and professional achievements. Assessing premorbid abilities is helpful in determining the degree of change that has occurred relative to the individual's original cognitive strengths and weaknesses.

Prevalence. The number of all new and old cases of a disease or condition in a defined population at a particular point in time. For example, the prevalence of MS in the United States at any given time is about 1/750—approximately 400,000 people.

Primary-progressive MS. *See* Disease course.

Procedural memory. The long-term memory of skill-based learning or "how-to" knowledge (e.g., how to walk, ride a bicycle, make a cake, throw a baseball) that becomes automatic with repetition. It is also often referred to as *"non-declarative" memory or "implicit memory."* Procedural memory and declarative memory together comprise what we think of as memory. *See* Declarative memory; Memory.

Progressive-relapsing MS (PRMS). *See* Disease course.

Recognition. The ability to recognize or identify information that has previously been stored in memory. It is usually assessed by presenting material that has been previously viewed, along with new material, and asking the individual to identify the previously-seen material.

Relapsing-remitting MS (RRMS). *See* Disease course

Retention. The ability to hold on to or remember information over time.

Retrograde memory. The recall of any information that was learned prior to disease onset or brain injury. *See* Anterograde memory.

Retrieval deficit. A memory problem characterized by the inability to recall information quickly and freely, without the benefit of the passage of time or additional cues.

Retrieval phase (of memory process). The phase of the memory process in which information that has been previously stored in the brain is accessed or recalled for current use.

Secondary-progressive MS (SPMS). *See* Disease course.

Semantic memory. The memory for general information and facts, including the recognition and meaning of words, objects, actions, and facts that are not tied to specific time and place of learning (e.g., the meaning of vocabulary words). It is most often contrasted with episodic memory, which refers to the recall of events. Semantic and episodic memory together comprise declarative memory. *See* Declarative memory; Episodic memory.

Speech/language pathologist (SPL). A health care professional who specializes in the diagnosis and treatment of speech and swallowing disorders. A person with MS may be referred to a speech/language pathologist for help with either one or both of these problems. Because of their expertise with speech and language difficulties, these specialists also provide cognitive remediation for individuals with cognitive impairment.

Storage deficit. A memory problem characterized by the inability to consolidate information in a meaningful way for subsequent retrieval. A person with a storage deficit cannot recall or recognize materials once his or her attention has been removed from it.

U.S. Food and Drug Administration (FDA). The U.S. federal agency that is responsible for enforcing governmental regulations pertaining to the manufacture and sale of food, drugs, and cosmetics. Its role is to prevent the sale of impure or dangerous substances. Any new drug that is proposed for the treatment of MS in the United States must be approved by the FDA.

Verbal IQ. A composite score that summarizes the Verbal scale subtest scores obtained on a test battery measuring overall intellectual abilities (e.g., the Wechsler Adult Intelligence Scale [WAIS]). It is commonly considered a measure of verbal cognitive functioning and may be used to derive premorbid estimates. *See* Premorbid estimation.

Working memory. Previously called *"short-term memory,"* this term refers to the short-term storage (up to 15 or 20 seconds) of information, which can be maintained as long as it is continually rehearsed (e.g., repeating the telephone number that someone is giving you for as long as it takes you to write it on a piece of paper). Working memory also refers to the mental manipulation of briefly- stored information in order to solve a problem (e.g., how much change you should receive when purchasing an item) or organize information for memory recall.

INDEX